ENER

The Patterns & Techniques of
EmoTrance™
Vol. 3

Silvia Hartmann, PhD

First Paperback Edition 2006

ISBN 1 873483 767

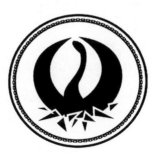

**Published By
DragonRising**

Energy Magic
The Patterns & Techniques of EmoTrance Volume 3
© Silvia Hartmann, PhD 2006

ISBN10 1-873483-76-7
ISBN13 978-1-873483-76-3

First Edition 2006

Published by:
DragonRising Publishing
18 Marlow Avenue
Eastbourne BN22 8SJ
United Kingdom
https://www.DragonRising.com

All Rights Reserved in all media, including future media.
Printed and bound by CPI Antony Rowe Ltd, Eastbourne

Other titles by Silvia Hartmann:

Oceans of Energy: The Patterns & Techniques of EmoTrance, Vol. 1
Living Energy: The Patterns & Techniques of EmoTrance, Vol. 2
Energy Magic: The Patterns & Techniques of EmoTrance, Vol. 3
Adventures in EFT: Your Essential Guide to Emotional Freedom
The Advanced Patterns of EFT
EFT & NLP
Project Sanctuary
For You, A Star: Essential Magic for Every Day
The Enchanted World
MindMillion
EmoTrance Practitioner: Correspondence Training Programme
Meridian Energy Therapy Practitioner (AMT Prac): Correspondence Training Programme
The Story Teller: Correspondence Training Programme
Energy Healing For Animals: Correspondence Training Programme
The In Serein Trilogy
Vampire Solstice

EDITORIAL NOTES

In compiling this first edition of "Energy Magic – The Patterns & Techniques of EmoTrance, Volume 3" it has been attempted to preserve as much of Dr Silvia Hartmann's unique style of presentation as possible. The main body of material is a direct transcript which remains essentially unedited as well as uncensored; only direct product references have been replaced.

During the lectures, occasions arose where Dr Hartmann delivered hypnotic inductions for the audience. These have been line broken so that a reader may recognise these events.

We hope that in the production of this edition we have succeeded in allowing Dr Silvia Hartmann's voice and energy to carry across from the spoken word to the written pages, so that the contact between the author and the reader is preserved.

The Editorial Team,

DragonRising Publishing

November 2005

Acknowledgements

We thank the following for their support in developing this material.

The primary research team:
Nicola Quinn
Steve Collins

Also acknowledged are:
Alex Kent
Ananga Sivyer
The Heros Team

TABLE OF CONTENTS

EDITORIAL NOTES 3

ACKNOWLEDGEMENTS 5

PART 1 11

The EmoTrance Journey, So Far 13

Art Solutions Revisited 15
  The Bottled Energetic Reality 15
  The Art Solutions Set Up 17

The Pleasure/More Pleasure Principle 18
  Magic Here, And Now 23
  Ingesting Energy Food 25
  Flexible Responses 25

The Art Of Symbol Making 27
  Introducing The Marps 28
  Symbols As Movements 32
  Potion Making 34

Healing With Plant Energy 36

PART 2 37

Healing With Plant Energy (continued) 39
  Plant Energy & EmoTrance 39

The Planes Concept 42
  The Conscious Concentration Camp 43

A Matter Of Fear 48
  Fear Creates Poisons 53

Magic & Luck 58
  The Auspicious Time Exercise 60

Custom Rituals 64
  An Exercise In Movement 71

PART 3 73

Custom Rituals (continued) 75
The Spirit Of The Thing 75

Symbols & Structural Integrity 77
Focus On Structure, Not Effect 82
Money Injury Exercise 85
Life Raft On The Sea Of Details 87

Directional Affirmations and Magic Spells 89
Human Will & Reality Creation 91
The Celtic House Warming Snail 94

Who Do You Want To Be 97
Wish Fulfilment To Unlock Incarnations 99

PART 4 101

The Duty To Make Dreams Come True 103
Discipline 105

Magic Affirmations 108
Crocodiles VS Golden Horses 113
Freedom Spells & Totality Goals 117

Energy Dancing 119
Loving Yourself 126

ADDENDUM 1 135

Project Energy 137
Welcome To Project Energy! 137
Your Idea 138
The Dissonance Factor 139
Calibrating The Energy Of A Project 140
Genesis – THE IDEA 142
Important Notes On The Threshold Challenge 145
The Project Energy 147
Your First Unique Project Energy 149
You & Your Project 151
The Magical Project Feedback Mechanisms 152
Problems With The Project 152
Fine Tuning Your Project 154
The Project Identity 155
The Project Messengers 157

Attracting The Right Energies In Return 158
The Naming Ceremony 159
Assistance, Guidance and Conditions 164
Recipients & Facilitators 164
Project Adjustments 166
Getting Practical 170
The Journey Has Begun ... .174
Project Energy Conclusion – And Some Metaphysical Musings 175

EmoTrance To Energy Magic: The Freedom Spells 177
The Spell Format 177
Freedom Spells The Basic Instructions 178
Freedom Spells - Examples 179

Comments On The Freedom Spells 186
Releasing Questions 187
PS - A Brief Note On Using Freedom Spells With Clients 189

BeauTy T – Healing The Shattered Body Image 190
Beauty T – A General Introduction 190
Back To BeauTy Basics 192
What is Beauty T? 193
The Process of Beauty T 193
Benefits Of Beauty T For The Client 194
Beauty T Self Help 196
The Client Practitioner Dance 198
Beauty T As A Major Benefit For EmoTrance Clients 199
Beauty T PinPoint 200
Charging For Beauty T 201
BeauTy T – Example Wording 202
BeauTy T - In Conclusion 210

BeauTy T For Animals 211
BeauTy T For Animals 211

Energy Magic: Creating A Powerful Training Ritual 214
Order & Sequence In The Ritual 216
Free Talismans 217
The Ritual Surround 217
A First True Magical Ritual 220

Magic Words 222
Quick Power Words Exercises 224

The Golden Line 225
   Peers & Repayments 226
   The Hero Transaction..227
   A Unique Repayment 228

EmoTrance – The Resolution 230

ADDENDUM 2 - FURTHER INFORMATION 232

   About The Author 232
   About DragonRising 238

Part 1

The EmoTrance Journey, So Far ...

Good Morning, Ladies & Gentlemen!

And what a lovely day it is today.

The sun is shining, the birds are singing - somewhere. Just a few kilometres up, no more than one or two, the sun is shining permanently. Yes, it is, above the clouds. It's really amazing when you go up in an airplane from a day like this or when it's pouring with rain, you go up and up and up, and for a while you see nothing at all, and then – sunshine! Which is a very nice thing indeed and a nice thing to remember once in a while.

Well, well, well my friends! How delightful to see you here this morning. I have seen many of you many times before, and the more I see you, the more I like you. Strange, that, but it's quite wonderful really.

Now, this day marks actually quite an important event in my calendar in so far as this is the end of the EmoTrance journey. Isn't that great? This journey began some time in 2002 with EmoTrance Level 1 and that amazing event in Kensington. There, we had the astonishing insight that the emotions are actually feedback mechanisms from the energy body, which is quite remarkable that it should have escaped humanity for the last few hundred thousand years. We started playing and working with that and using this to get a completely different handle I would say on our own emotions.

Before, it was this huge big thing, wasn't it.

My fear, my pain, my shame, my guilt and it was just "It's only an energy!" My burden, my weight, my broken heart – "It's only an energy!" Stop bitching, will you. Heal that, repair that, do something with it.

Which for me personally was absolutely marvellous, because I didn't like going round wailing, "Booohoohoo, my mother mistreated me when I was three years old ..." I was so tired of it. Because it didn't do anything, either. You can do this forever and ever and it doesn't do anything. And the other thing I really like about it is this confluence of what I call love and logic, where emotions become logical, and Mr Spock is once more on board, and is learning to sing and beginning to explore his own emotions without being afraid of them. This is a very nice thing indeed.

I love it when people go to a basic EmoTrance training and they say, "I came here and I was going to sit here and pluck it all apart consciously as I do at all the trainings I attend, but – damn it! This is actually logical, it's reasonable, it is scientific. I shall have to believe it ..."

So, that was EmoTrance 1, and jolly good fun it was too, and is being used by a great many people in a great many ways to get over old emotional problems, to open the door to a new life which is really what we need.

We need to turn away from the past and focus on the future, because only the future has the experiences which we haven't yet had, but we jolly well want to have, even need to have in order to actualise our own personal immortality.

Which brings me to EmoTrance 2, Living Energy.

Whilst we were working with the energy system in the way that we do as EmoTrance practitioners, we found out some really interesting things as to how emotion, energy, thought, behaviour and thus actualised reality is being created. We came across the marvel of the autogenic universe, the matrix, and we found out that we as human beings have this amazing capability to imbue things with energy realities behind the scenes.

We learned that we could do things such as turning a little jelly bean into a magical device for goal setting, or a plain glass into a healing chalice by working with the energetic realities behind the scenes. And that was very exciting, was it not?

And it is exciting, because I still do this every day. I check things for the existing energetic realities behind, and if I don't like them, I change them or replace the objects, which is a wonderful thing to be able to do.

Right at the end of EmoTrance 2, there comes another paradigm shifter and you might have heard of this before, and this is the place at which we bridge from ET2 into ET3.

This paradigm shifter was Art Solutions.

Art Solutions Revisited

The Bottled Energetic Reality

Just briefly to remind ourselves, as we were working with the energetic realities and effect behinds behind visible or hard objects, we came across things like The Scream, by Edward Munch.

That's a picture where someone stands on a bridge and has clearly had it with the world and goes, "Aaaargh, my God!"

Now, we called that "a bottled energetic reality" because the artist managed to capture this energy in a canvas, and even when this image is being photocopied, or made into a poster and it is no longer the original, the energy goes with it. A poster of the scream on the bedroom wall of a suicidal person can easily lead them to enter into a feedback loop with their own and his pain, winding itself up tighter and faster and harder until the point when they jump of a cliff comes.

Now, this is not what our friend Edvard Munch ever wanted. If he wanted people to jump off a cliff, then it would have been the ones that caused the screams in the first place, not those who were screaming, like himself. So something happened there that this poor man never really foresaw. But in the days when he was painting this, images were not as easily transmissible as they are today. You would have had to have made an art print of this which would have been quite difficult in those days. Now we have the internet and such images can be anywhere, and they are, and they *still* scream, all the time.

I have an aspect of me who is an artist and a lot of my friends are artists too, and we began to realise that we had been painting our own screams, sculpting and writing and singing our own screams, and thus effectively contributing to the misery in the world.

We did this because we thought that this is what artists have to do. You honestly go to your honest emotions, your honest energy of what you're feeling and then you throw all of that, bleeaurch, like a sea cucumber who will puke out its guts. That's what art is. And a work of art is when people come up and they see it, and they throw up as well, and then everyone is delighted, because that's what art is all about, ***to get a response.***

Those are desperate measures. We came up with the idea to use art slightly more ecologically and holistically, because if we can create energetic realities which can be bottled and passed on through generations, I believe the Adagio in G Minor by Albinoni was written in the 15th century. How many people have cried their eyes out over that thing since then? How many performances? It's a very powerful thing, isn't it, it's really quite amazing. So we thought, how can we turn this around and make a POSITIVE CONTRIBUTION if any, as artists, as human beings, I really do not wish to increase the misery that already exists on this planet.

There was a time when I wanted to increase the misery on the grounds that I was very angry and wanted other people to suffer as much as I did.

Since then I've come to the conclusion that people already suffer plenty and I find it hard to come up with any ideas to make them suffer even more than they already do. To many, a good flogging with clean pain would be a relief because it would take their minds off the churning nastiness that resides in their lives in general.

So I thought, I'll find another way to take revenge at another time and see if I can contribute something positive. And the question arose as how to do that. It was as simple as asking for a solution instead of puking your pain onto the canvass, the piano, the writing keyboard or through the quill, to simply stop and say, "Ok, so I feel like that – aaaargh! – but now, energy mind, give me a SOLUTION for this."

Guess what happened?

Well it did.

It wasn't a matter of having to do a deep trance induction, or to do anything really. It was simply a question to ask for a solution to be given and to step back and see what happens next.

So I'm going to put Art Solutions right at the top now, because although it comes from art, I don't want you to sit there and think to yourself, "It has nothing to do with me, I'm not an artist," for it has, and you are.

The Art Solutions Set Up

The Art Solution set up is as simple as saying, "Give me some thing ... to ...."

Some of the applications for that are just hinted at the end of EmoTrance 2, Living Energy. You could stand in front of your fridge and say, "Give me something out of all the choices here for me to be eating, or having or ingesting, right now."

It's interesting that people don't do that. It is an application of consciousness. Normally, if you are peckish you go to the fridge, you open the door, you reach inside, take the first thing and you eat it. Or if you are used to that first thing always being a certain kind of thing, such as ice cream or cheese, or chocolate, or whatever it is, we just keep doing these sort of things over and over again, and they will keep running until somebody says, "Stop! We're doing something else!"

Now, unless that something is MORE PLEASURABLE, a BETTER choice, pleasurable, we're not going to do it.

So this is where you can't say to someone who has weight problems, choose between a salad leaf and a tub of your favourite Häagen-Daz. That is not a choice, BF Skinner even said that isn't a choice. In order to get away from the Häagen-Daz, you have to find something **more** pleasurable than the Häagen-Daz, not less pleasurable. Then you get away from it, and you get immediately away from it, one time learning, immediately, instantly, without any willpower and without ever looking back.

See this is where people switch from Marijuana to Speed, to Cocaine, to Heroin, and why it's so difficult to get them from Heroin to Methadone. That's not more pleasurable, it's shit in comparison. This is what makes it so hard.

The Pleasure/More Pleasure Principle

Our systems are DESIGNED to seek the <u>HIGHEST</u> PLEASURES.

We got that from the universe, the lord of the universe itself gave us this life and built it into us structurally to always seek the highest pleasure, the best experience, the cleanest water, the juiciest berry, the most gorgeous mate. It is built into all of us. Every one of us, even grasses and things, they try to creep over to where the soil is a little bit more nourishing. And they do.

Isn't that the most amazing thing?

Where people go wrong and where they make it so hard for themselves is that they try to replace something that is pleasurable and serves a purpose, with something that isn't and doesn't.

So it becomes very difficult to convince ourselves to eat a lettuce leaf when Häagen-Daz is such a fabulous experience and completely satisfies the need and the desire that we had for doing that. It becomes a lifelong uphill battle and nasty evil struggle and that's just a metaphor.

Those of you who are skinny as rakes, don't you dare sit there and think, "Tehehe ...!" No. You have your own battles and struggles with your own things that you don't seem to be able to overcome. And the reason is very simply that you need to replace the thing you want to get rid of *with something **MORE** pleasurable*.

It's a simple principle.

Now then.

Pleasure doesn't come from the mind.

Pleasure is a whole body experience.

Pleasure is something that you FEEL.

Feel it in your fingertips, you feel it in the tip of your tongue.

You feel it in your energy system, feel little shivers going down your spine and you go, "Oooh ..."

Just so we know what pleasure is.

It's a whole body experience, and a whole body experience involves, as we know from ET2,

- the conscious mind,
- the energy mind,
- the energy body,
- and the physical body,

all **together <u>at the same time.</u>**

In fact you could say whenever all of them are in the same place at the same time, pleasure ensues.

You could also say the inverse which is if any one of them is absent, it's not going to be very pleasurable.

It is impossible to feel real pleasure if your energy system is on reversal; it is impossible to feel real pleasure if your body has been disconnected; and it is impossible to feel pleasure if these two are having fun but you are thinking in your head that you should be ashamed of yourself and you're going to hell.

As I have just defined as pleasure as whole person state, they are quite different pleasures which are extremely pleasurable beyond Häagen-Daz, and I apologise to the company who makes this luscious thing, for using them as an example and I would encourage those who like Häagen-Daz to eat as much as you like of it. By denying yourself, you only create a worse and worse problem. But hopefully, we can do something for our all over totality health this way.

Let me remind you of a time when you were feeling inordinate pleasure.

Now this may have been when you were in a Jacuzzi, relaxing, feeling the nice hot water bubbling, everything was just well with the world and you were floating there, going "Aaaah ..."

It could have been on a sandy beach, or even on a stony beach. Nice fresh air, squawk, squawk, go the seagulls and you're thinking, "Oh yes! This is nice!"

Could be on a mountain top, or a family gathering, it matters not, really – but these are examples of pleasures beyond sitting sadly at your kitchen table feeling ashamed of yourself with a tub of Häagen-Daz.

That's the kind of pleasures we want to be aiming for. And the thing is that if you get yourself together with all your aspects, you can have such pleasures in front of your own fridge with for example a small raspberry. But that only happens if the mind, and the body, and the energy mind and the physicality are all in agreement that they want to eat this goddamned raspberry and that's the key of Art Solutions.

When you stand in front of your fridge and you have a reasonable selection of items inside, not the sort of thing you classically see in the movies where the cop is drinking and the wife has left him, and he opens the fridge and you know what he sees inside.

We don't want that. We want a reasonably well stocked fridge in our internal representations; two, three sorts of vegetables, some meat, some cheese, some interesting items; we stand in front of this and stand there as a totality, and we ask the art solutions question, "Give me something that gives me pleasure, right now." Then we see where the marps or the hands go, what they pick out. And if this just happens to be a small slice of cucumber, which, oldfashionedly you would not have picked, but on this occasion, in this moment, in this instant is just fantastic?

Where do I feel this in my body? Oh my God – where don't I? Cold, slightly stale – oooh, fantastic!

This is a different definition of pleasure, but you know this can be done, don't you?

You've had experiences of this. That something as simple as a glass of water at the right moment becomes a real orgasm, the best thing you've ever drank, beating the most expensive wine that's been lying at the bottom of the ocean for sixty years hands down because it was so cool.

I had one of those with plain orange juice the other day. I was really thirsty and in the right frame of mind, I went at this orange juice like a connoisseur would and had the most marvellous experience of it.

We have had experiences of this, and the fridge example is just one thing - we can take this a step back.

We can stand in a supermarket and say, "Show me what I need, what I want, to make me feel better, to make me happy, to experience ... PLEASURE!"

Just see what you buy!

It's very interesting, and it's very different from what you were used to having bought.

So, guys, think PLEASURE.

This goes for all kinds of decisions you make such as what clothes you are going to wear, what clothes you are going buy.

What television programmes you are going watch.

Asking the question of the totality as you're looking through the TV listings, "Give me something that gives me pleasure – NOW!"

The "now" at the end is not just a Bandler word.

Right NOW, Right HERE, as a flowing ecology, that's the thing, isn't it?

In 1963, Daddy bought this woman an ice cream, and she ate it on the beach. She's been eating that ice cream since 1963, regardless of whether her body wanted this ice cream, needed this ice cream, or anything.

This is like prescribing the same remedy all those years. That's a long time, 41 years. Imagine you took a remedy for 41 years for a problem that you had 41 years ago. This is what we're all doing with the things that we're using to keep our old Guiding Star/Trauma systems in place – we're not responding to the here and now as we should.

So, I want to write the word PLEASURE here:

PLEASURE

And pleasure isn't sin. Pleasure is what we were born to feel, and it isn't just about luxurious silks, it's about everything. It is an experience of some thing that is right for you at that moment in time.

So the next word is:

HERE AND NOW

This is very important.

Here and now. We can't heal the emotional problem we have right now with the remedy from 1963.

That's the last time that worked.

That is the ONLY time that worked, because that was the ONLY situation for which it was completely appropriate.

The key to pleasure, real living, living to the here and now, and responding adequately, correctly to the environments to find yourselves in, is to respond to what is there, and not what isn't.

That's pretty obvious, isn't it.

When we used to go shopping before I gave this talk, we used to be buying things and responding to things that happened way back when, like what mummy always bought, or what the husband used to like yesterday.

And he likes that because his mummy bought him that when he fell down and scraped his knee, in 1912.

Now that is no way to run a healthy body.

People have tried to get past this by blanket bombing.

"You need to eat 8 portions of vegetables a day."

That's the equivalent of the EFT protocol, for the love of God. You tap all the points and you get the right one by default.

So you eat 8 portions of vegetables a day, blanket bombing, to get that one tiny bit from one of these vegetables, and then only a tiny amount. So you needn't have chugged your way through all that god-damned broccoli that didn't give you pleasure on this day, because you didn't need it, you didn't want it, and there were parts of you that just went, "Bleargh!"

So we grimly stuff these vegetables down us because it's supposed to be good for us – "Bleaaaaargh!"

What kind of life is that?

My God!

Every other meal, it's a nightmare!

It's got to stop!

We've got to enjoy our food completely, it's got to give us total pleasure.

Magic Here, And Now

An American NLP trainer finally found his way to EmoTrance 1. He bought the book online as an eBook, downloaded it, read it whilst having his dinner. It occurred to him that he might be able to feel that hot chip in his mouth, and he did an EmoTrance on that hot chip in his mouth, the saltiness of it, and the guy nearly came!

The stuff just flowed through his body, through his energy system, and he was good with energy, so it really flowed and he went, "OH MY GOD!" He was completely overwhelmed with that.

And the other thing was that he actually didn't finish his plate of chips.

How many of "those" sort of chips can you eat before you lie on the floor and cry, and say, "Oh please! No more! I just can't take any more pleasure! Oh stop! Oh please stop!"

But it is actually true, once you have these whole body experiences with food, it does fill some thing, some where along the line, it becomes this totally different thing and it can't be compared to normal eating.

But the important thing is the response to here and now.

That is the key to magic, and it is:

Magic IS here and now.

It is not in the past, it's not in the future, it is HERE AND NOW.

Things happen as if by magic.

And magic has got to be PLEASURE.

It has GOT to be.

We are pleasure-designed beings.

Not the "pleasure/pain principle", that isn't true. We are organised ONLY by pleasure. The best thing, the brightest star, the tastiest fruit. That is what guides us to our decisions. Past traumas, they don't even compare.

Someone falls in love, it doesn't matter how many times they've been beaten with a stick by someone who looked just the same, they'll still marry them.

Which in and of itself is complete proof that those who think that people are driven by pain ARE WRONG.

People do not learn by pain. People do not get to learn how to be better people by pain. People do not lose weight by pain. People do not become healthier by pain. They can only have all these things BY PLEASURE.

The greater the pleasure, the greater the GAIN.

The bigger the Guiding Star, the happier your life, and the more magic you can get your hands on.

I can't say it any clearer than that.

How do you like that?

It sounds good?

When it really FEELS good, we'll be getting there.

>> Food Experience Exercise

Now, has everyone here got a small piece of food upon them?

I'd like you to try this as an EmoTrance exercise. We don't have any hot, salty chips, but you use whatever pathetic little mint, weasely sweet or chewing gum you have upon your person.

Hold on! This is an exercise. Don't start having pleasure just yet. Can't have too much pleasure – just wait ... wait there a little while longer. Let me tease you a little while longer before I allow you do this exercise. What I want you to do – in a moment! – is to place this thing into your mouth, put your attention into the whole act of eating this. Put any conscious objections on hold – eeouwh, this is making me fat! Eeeouwh, this is bad for my teeth, eeeeouwh ... Just tell it to shut up.

Experience this. Let the energy radiate throughout you.

Do it – right now!

Ingesting Energy Food

Ok, let the eating stop now.

Perhaps we should call it "ingesting" or something else instead ...

Someone offered me a rock solid hard mint to try. I was not in the mood to crunch into that so I put it in my hand instead and pulled the energy through and came across quite a remarkable energy blockage in my neck that hurt quite badly when the mint energy hit it. I got to resolve that so that is a good thing but it's nice to remind us that if we want the energy of an object, we don't have to eat it.

That was fun, wasn't it?

So go and change your shopping habits.

It's a super exercise because it reminds us of **instant response** rather than responding to the old. Most people live their life on old stimuli. Their decisions are all based on old traumas and old Guiding Stars, not really what they need here and now.

Once you change that ...

You need to change that if you want change, if you want to change lives, change your life, have more pleasure in it, have more health in it, have more fulfilment in it. We need to be more flexible.

Flexible Responses

"Light on your feet must you be ..."

That's in my magic dedication. It also says that "magic sings and dances" – it is LIGHT. That's why you can't confine it with symbols, heavy with metal, heavy with age.

Now then.

"Give me something to ..."

We've had the very simplest level there – something to watch, something to eat, something to feel, something to experience, and at the far end we have the art solutions proper.

This is where a pianist says, "Give me something to heal that old pain that I've been writing the same old song about in A minor since I first started composing when I was 13."

What then happens is that for someone who can play the piano, their hands just go and they produce a melody.

When they produce that melody, the person who is producing that melody is sitting back in shock and astonishment, and says, "Oh my God, that is so beautiful! That is just so amazing! I didn't know I could make music like that! And it – feels so GOOD!"

Yes, it would, wouldn't it, darling.

Because it is a SOLUTION not a re-statement of the old problem, over and over again.

I personally am quite good with the old keyboard, as in with letters and words, so I ask the question of, "Give me something to make me feel better tonight." And then, I get a poem or something, if I remember on one point, even a Haiku.

That really annoyed me, because it reminded me of the old grasshopper thing.

"Master, can you help me please? I am really confused!"

"Well now, Grasshopper. The cow stares into the mirrored pond once more and the swallows fly up in the hills."

"Yes ... thank you master ... that was very helpful ..."

Art solutions are good fun.

You can do mashed potato shapes if you want to.

Don't think you can't do this. Of course you can!

If you can ask what should I eat right now, and your attention is drawn to a particular thing in your fridge then your attention can be called to a single key on your keyboard; it can be called to a single colour, to a single line or even to a single movement.

And one of the wonderful things we are going to do this morning is ...

The Art Of Symbol Making

Do you know Reiki symbols?

I saw one once that made me nearly throw up.

Some woman made it, some Reiki woman made that thing and I thought, if other people use this symbol, they'll all get YOUR womb cancer!

It was like that, very idiosyncratic.

A scream, rather than an art solution.

If you make a magical symbol from a state of disturbance, what do you get?

You get a scream!

Would you be surprised if I told you if 99% of all symbols in use are screams, rather than solutions?

99.9% of magic rituals are screams, rather than solutions.

It's true.

But we can do better than that, which is very nice.

Introducing The Marps

So this is a very nice exercise we are all going to do as a group, right now.

Please put your things away and rise to your pretty feet.

Those of you who were at Eastbourne last year, you will already know all about marps.

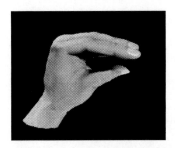

This is a marp.

Have you all got one?

Say "Hello!" to your marp, and your marp says back, "Marp, marp!"

And you don't have just one, you have two.

Say "Hello!" to the second one too.

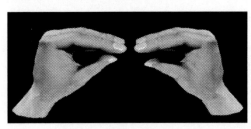

And please apologise to the second marp for not calling him first, assure him that he is equally beloved. Kiss him briefly on the snout and notice how the marp is joyous when you do that.

Now, marps are quite interesting because they have a bit of a life of their own. And of course, and for the people who don't know about marps, there are evil marps.

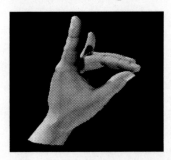

Make an evil marp.

It's quite simply, let me demonstrate how a marp gets to be evil.

You have a nice ordinary marp, and if you strike it, like this, it turns evil.

Now, it is evil, but if you stroke the horns quite gently, it becomes nice again and you have a normal marp once more.

That's great.

When we do art solutions that involve pointing, painting, writing, or making movements of any kind, or even sometimes shopping, it's quite helpful to think of giving over the control of the choice to your marp.

When you say to people "Let your hand do it," it just doesn't work that way.

My hands, they are waiting for instructions from me, of course they would, but marps, they can act independently.

On this occasion, we shall use the marp you are most familiar with, and we are going to use this marp to let us draw a little symbol of health.

Imagine you were standing in front of a canvas and the marp was holding a small, gentle wax crayon that glides easily, and we are going to ask the marp to draw us a little symbol of health.

You can do this with your eyes open or with your eyes shut.

Just let your marp draw your symbol, something that you need, right now.

Ok, everybody got one?

Are the marps co-operating?

Do it a few more times to get the shape of that symbol fixed in consciousness so that you can repeat it if someone asked you to show it to you.

Ah, very good.

So we have all got a symbol for health, in the here and now?

Then you may take a seat, and thank your marp. Do it meaningfully! Marps like to be appreciated and it helps with their co-operation with more complex projects in the future.

Would you like to show me your symbol for health?

Just let your marp do it. Do it again. Ok, can you draw it on your papers now? Draw it down.

I remember mine.

Here it is:

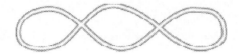

I thought that was quite neat. I was following it along in some fascination.

Now, if I was a Japanese Reiki master, I would have you all make this one. But what good would that do anyone? You don't have MY bizarre on goings, you are not ME.

That wouldn't help anyone at all.

- **You have to MAKE YOUR OWN SYMBOLS for magic, for life – you have to make your own symbols, your own rituals, your own magic.**

This is what we are learning here today, for you to make your own decisions and pathways, in accordance with the rules of the universe, with the laws of creation, and so that it always feels really, really good.

Now, when you look at that symbol you made, how does that feel?

Yours, not mine.

It feels nice? Where do you feel that energy in your body?

Is this pleasant? Interesting?

Do we have any "non-creative" people here who have a nice little symbol?

See look, the applications for this are truly endless.

Imagine, I wanted to open a health clinic and I needed a symbol.

Well, there it is.

Imagine I wanted to design a special T Shirt that I will wear when I go to sleep to help me with my health magically, that will support my energy system when I'm too tired and too knackered to do EmoTrance, and I have no reserves left.

I could put that symbol on such a T Shirt.

I could use that symbol for a springboard for inspiration of all kinds – for patterns, for dance, for music, for behaviour, for all sorts.

It is as simple as letting the marp do it, ASKING the marp to do it.

As simple as that.

Try this one. You can stay sitting for this one.

"Give me a small symbol AGAINST FEAR."

You can do it straight on the pad if your marp is willing, if not, draw it in the air first a few times before you've got it down.

Are we making magic yet?

When you are doing this, you mustn't think about it, you must let the marp do it. YOU just get to watch.

I can see in the audience that people are getting a real energy kick. Isn't this great?

By the way, if your marp freezes up when you give him a pen and he freezes up and just becomes a hand again, take the pen away, give him a little kiss and let him do the symbol in the air.

This is the very simplest form of symbol making.

It is based on the art solutions questions of, "Give me something FOR ..."

"Give me something that does ..."

"Give me something that heals that ..."

Also, you could say:

"Give me something – for Sandra."

If you do this for others, it is really easy to ask, "Give me a symbol for Sandra."

I personally make business logos this way and it is true that my businesses are always energetically very interesting.

"Give me a symbol for success ..."

Symbols As Movements

Now what we are going to do later is that we are going to dance this and get the whole body involved, and make BIG symbols.

Not just little piddly ones. Have you ever heard about submodalities? The smaller something is, the less excited you get about it.

Big submodalities, big things.

If you want to create big realities and you want to experience big energy shifts, the symbols become a great deal bigger.

However, and as this is a course in magic, and how to make your own magic, this is how symbols are made; this is how you can make your own book of symbols, for all sorts of reasons and all sorts of purposes, but what I would much prefer is if you didn't.

In fact if any of you should go out and start to make books of symbols and tell everyone they're the same and sell them, my spirit will come to haunt you.

- **You see, it's the act of MAKING THE SYMBOLS that we learn how we respond to ourselves and we get our whole totality working together – the head and the mind and the body and the energy system.**

It's a wonderful thing.

It is the MOVEMENT IN A SYMBOL which actually energises the energy flow in the energy body.

It is NOT a line on a piece of a paper, but it really is a **MOVEMENT.**

Do you understand that?

Good.

What else can we do with that little skill of making symbols at will, purposefully, deliberately, with every malice of forethought?

"Give me a symbol for my new business, that will encompass my mission, and will be immensely successful as well as bringing those people to me who I want the most, and who will give me the most pleasure."

See, the energy mind is a clever, clever little bastard.

I've got to tell you this.

DON'T think that you can only ask simple little kiddie question such as give me a symbol for health right now.

You can make this as complicated as you want, and I have proof of this.

I got a list of 250 search engine question terms ...

<Audience Member: It was 300.>

Ok, so 300.

300 separate phrases and terms people have typed into their search engines to find information on metaphor:

- Metaphor Poem,
- Metaphor Poems,
- Poems with Metaphor,

... and so on. The top 300. I said to my energy mind, "Right. Write me an article that contains all of these in order and sequence, that is good enough to be interesting and educational for a young schoolchild to understand what metaphor is so they can please their teachers, yet at the same time, delights advanced NLP trainers, that'll be fun to read, completely useful and from which I will learn something myself."

And the marps started to type, and you can find that article on The Sidereus Foundation. It's fabulous, and it contains all 300 search terms in order, one after the other, inside of it.

It did this, whoom, just like that.

So you can stipulate all sorts of outcomes onto a single symbol.

Consciously we can't do this.

Consciously, we can't even make symbols.

Real symbols are only unconsciously derived – of course! The energy mind is the guy who knows about energy and how to translate that into forms, shapes and movements. Every letter is a movement. Japanese calligraphy is a movement. Sword play is the same movement. Healing symbols are the same movement. Stroking your lover is the same movement.

This is a general rule of the Universe – movement.

Now that was easy and fun, wasn't it?

Was that worth your course fee so far? Yes?

Cool. So we can play for the rest of the day now we've got that over with.

Potion Making

In the advertising it said we would learn how to make potions, right?

Have a little think.

You are standing in front of a cupboard, containing a number of Bach Flower remedies.

How do we use the art solutions process to pick the right ones for a complex problem we have, right now?

Of course.

It's exactly the same as standing in front of your fridge.

"Give me something to heal that problem I have with my ex husband," and just let the marp loose on it.

At the beginning, you can just play cold, warm, hot.

Is it this one?

No, no, no ... hm, perhaps ... aha! This one!

JUST this single one?

That way, you get some fabulous potions that really work for you.

It doesn't matter if you use bat's tails, homeopathy, fruit juice, or crystals, or a mixture thereof. It's a wonderful process, it's good fun and you know when you get it right.

That way, you get things that actually work for you, rather than things which don't.

And the most important thing about the magic is that there is no delay.

No delay on the pleasure.

This is why they call it magic, and they don't understand how it works.

You give someone a headache tablet, it takes four hours for it to take effects.

But if you make a symbol, it is INSTANT.

How is that possible?!

Structurally, the blood vessels are still constricted, bla bla and serotonin bla bla ...

Well yes, that's why they call it MAGIC.

Because it isn't like *that*, but like THIS instead.

Now, we can make potions.

We can choose colours.

We can make symbols.

What else could magic possibly be?

And that's a lovely question, and a question we can take into the break with us.

Healing With Plant Energy

Those of you who want to go for a quick walk around the garden, I have an interesting little exercise you can try.

Imagine you were indigenous to this part of the world, and that the plants in this garden are *all there is*.

So your healing plant will have to come from this garden.

What it is that you have to take home and make yourself a brew out of that will help you the best with the problem you've got?

You'll find one. Don't eat it, just suck the energy into yourself.

So you get to try this principle.

What this is is actually directly READING the plants, the minerals, the whole thing what is good for you and what isn't.

That way, you get to make the potions.

You don't look them up in a book that some German wrote 200 years ago. Here and now, totally specific, highly complex and JUST FOR YOU.

You will find something in the garden. Simply pull the energy into yourself and it will make a significant difference to how good you feel – that's the key, how YOU FEEL.

That's how you KNOW the difference.

PART 2

Healing With Plant Energy (continued)

Plant Energy & EmoTrance

Did you find an indigenous plant to help you?

Well, I did. It was good. It is quite cool to do the exercises yourself as well. It's nice.

I found some variegated ivy and it wasn't quite right, it's an interesting sensation, a feedback device when it's nearly there but not quite. And we all know what that feels like. It's possibly even more frustrating than not at all, really. I thought, "Hm, I don't know, that's not it ..." wandered along a bit and noticed some non-variegated ivy, and that did the trick.

When I took the energy inside it actually impacted interestingly enough the back of my legs, the back of my calves and in the small of my back, which are the places which I usually have trouble with after standing up and talking all day. Not yet, because it's still early, but by five o'clock I notice this, and when I am home and get in the bath, that's the places where I store my stress. It's quite interesting that this should happen this morning there. I thought, "That's interesting, I shall visit the ivy again in the next break." I have some confidence that I will be able to conduct this whole day and not experience this slight soreness from standing.

Self medication using indigenous plants, so we don't have to import Kala Kala juice which is only found in a small insect in the desert of Nevada. There are things in this environment which can help us quite nicely.

I know a gentleman who wrote a book called The Herbal First Aid Kit. It has these 15 superherbs in them as he calls it, and they are not at all Ginseng or anything like that – they are parsley and onion, things we all really have, and it's just a wonderful thing to not just be able to use the highest forms of esoteric magic, which we will get to this afternoon, but also good old kitchen magic in one and the same system.

That brings together the male and female, the ying and the yang, because traditionally the women do the kitchen magic with the herbs and the men do the esoteric magic with the symbols and the alchemy.

This system makes no distinction between them, it's one and the same thing, which makes it very powerful – apart from the fact that you are using it individually for yourself, and not on behalf of anyone else, which makes it even more powerful still, and that's really rather neat. It's a politically correct system, if you will.

It is also completely independent of any kind of tradition, or genetic heritage, or anything like that, because you are dealing directly with the world itself with your body and your energy mind; your conscious mind just has to learn to follow suit, get out of the way if necessary, to think the right thoughts and to support the actions of the others in the first place.

My definition of magic is when things work as they should.

Really. Not fish falling from the sky and flapping on the ground. Not great big demons manifesting and going "Whoooo ..."

Real magic is when things work as they should, or even better than they should. We had good fun with EmoTrance 2 with the autogenic universe when we realised that there was no word in the English language which denotes the opposite to disappoint. In fact, there is not only no opposite to disappointment, there is no middle point between disappointment, the opposite which we don't have. For example, you get good, neutral and bad. Disappointment is only bad, and the other two are completely missing from our language. You can get quite complicated and talk about my expectations having been met or exceeded, but that isn't it.

Disappointment is like being punched in the stomach, it's instant, it's not a mental thing, it's just a "Ooouwh!" or worst, so the opposite must exist as an energy movement, where you're experiencing, "Whooooah!" That would be – propointment?

Disappointment is a very specific thing, when something is not as good as you wanted it to be. I want something that is much better than we thought it was going to be and *there is no word for that*.

There is even no word for things being **exactly** like you wanted things to be. Like satisfaction, it is an interesting feeling, that middle one.

At one point I started this Internet portal and said that one day, it would have a million visitors. Nobody believed me, but it happened. There was this day last year when we were all sitting in the office looking at the visitor counting clicking off – 999 998, 999 999, ... ONE MILLION.

I just went, "Yes!"

That's a sort of appointment. I knew it was going to happen and it happened exactly as I said it would. But the other side of that is missing.

Which is exactly the problem with ideas about healing when the best outcome is the concept of peace as some form of ceiling, like when the the pain stops, that's health – and it's not.

That's just NOTHING, ZERO and the real healing and the real life and real fun is actually ON THE OTHER SIDE. It's not until we start we are doing some magic that we begin to realise how bloody miserable this muppet world is, and how appalling the presuppositions of pain and suffering, and the best you can ever get is that the pain doesn't get too bad ...

Oh my God, it's appalling! It is HORRENDOUS!

This brings me nicely to a very important concept that leads us into High Magic, into esoteric magic, which is the planes concept.

The Planes Concept

For many, many years, people have tried to work out the world. They have worked really hard. One of these people was Alister Crowley. He dedicated his entire life to work out how the universe works, and he wasn't very successful at it, I'm afraid.

This was really shown by his life, how it worked out and the state he was in at the end of it – he was not a happy bunny.

We decided at some point, last week it might have been, that the outcome of our endeavours should be to lie on our deathbeds, in a hospice, and to be completely SMUG.

Just lying there right, laughing to yourself, haha, ouch, cough, hahahaha, oh yeah, hahaha, I've had a great life ... haha .. ouw, cough ... haha ...

Something like that.

That would drive the other people crazy, wouldn't it. They'd have to wheel you into a corner and put curtains round you so they wouldn't have to look at you dying and being smug.

That's a good point to set as an outcome for your life, to lie on your deathbed and be feeling smug, because you've had these experiences, you've had a good life, a good time, a fucking good ride – as Jim Morrison said, "Is there enough of your life to base a movie on?"

ONE?

A million of them!

So, poor old Alister and many before him tried to work out how the universe works, and I think I have worked out where they went wrong. I love that. Seneca, Plato ... I'd love to have them here and discuss this with them.

But look, so we've got the natural order of things and this has universal laws. We are aware of this, we have ants, sunrises and so forth, and we have also a number of different planes of existence with different laws of nature.

So we've got the Hard, with gravity and backwards and forwards, left and right and all of that, and we've got the energy levels for example which have completely different laws of nature, which has confused many. Such as, thought is instantly here and there, and time is everywhere at the same time, holographic occurrences and all of that.

They have different laws of nature and they are quite predictable.

But then we have our lives as people, here.

And that's the problem.

We need to do this differently if we want to do magic properly.

We need to split it up differently.

The Conscious Concentration Camp

So, here we have God's universe of which we are a part, because we have bodies, energy systems and so forth, and this has these planes like physicality and the energy levels and many others besides that I can't know anything about, not until I am somewhere else, and someone else, and something else, but what we call the Hard has actually nothing to do with God at all.

It's a sort of a bizarre concentration camp that humans have built for themselves that doesn't actually follow the same rules as the rest of the universe at all.

It is a nonsensical, bizarre fucked up construct, and I can only use that term, completely fucked up, that has nothing to do with that lovely universe which we see outside our windows, with the beautiful sunsets, and the ants doing their stuff, and the zebras and the lions, and our own body and our own experiences of love and healing and all the rest of it with its universal laws, rules and regulations, and then we have the Hard which does NOT FOLLOW THOSE LAWS and regulations – the concentration camp *does not follow the natural order of things*.

The concentration camp is completely *man made*.

And I won't excuse the women from this. They may say that it wasn't them and that they didn't have a hand in this, but by God, they ALWAYS had a hand in it.

This thing, this blot on the universal landscape, is *human made*.

You could use another metaphor and call all of that outside PARADISE, and this is the valley of the shadows or we can just call it the concentration camp, or the Hard.

In the real universe, we find all the things that people really, really like on a deep, structural and visceral level, such as joy, love, justice, order, predictability, even in storm floods there is a predictability that they will come eventually if you sit for long enough next to an ocean.

Things being the way they are, things *being right*.

But in the Hard, which is this bizarre construct with toasters and garden gnomes, law books, poetry albums, EVERYTHING that people do, these *laws of nature are being attempted to be suspended or even contravened*.

It is a HUGE struggle to try and keep that up, it is a never ending struggle because it wants to collapse back all the time into the natural order of things – obviously.

If you are having difficulty conceptualising this, all you have to do is to look out the window at these GODAWFUL rose beds out there.

Those water logged sticks sticking out of the ground which have been grafted on some other thing, some travesties in squares that people have put there because they think that's BETTER THAN NATURE.

I could not give you a better example than that MISERY that is happening right outside that window, and which is known as a formal rose garden.

Madness like that does not exist in nature AT ALL.

This is where people have become confused. They have their own experiences of living in this concentration camp where people who lie and cheat get rewarded, and those who honestly try to do their best get kicked in the head.

You know that, don't you?

Where lies are bought and sold, where pain and suffering is bought and sold, where people get away with blue MURDER – and it doesn't make any sense, and then you look at the beautiful skies and the sunsets and you ask yourself, how can I put THESE together?

HOW can I make some kind of map that makes any kind of sense at all?

And the deal is that you can't put those together, and in trying, you will only make an INSANE MAP.

Aha!

So what we need to do and I will leave that to your energy minds, your unconscious minds, is to start unravelling the maps that you have made of "the world" and actually split it up into a number of projector foils, and understand that the local conventions in one are not the same as in the other, but most importantly, that **in the Hard, in our concentration camp, the local conventions do NOT follow the natural order of things.**

There, different things apply.

There, it is really true that justice doesn't rule the day, or that beauty triumphs – this concentration camp doesn't work like that.

But it DOES HAVE RULES – and we know exactly how they work, because each one of us has been brought up here.

We know the regulations of the concentration camp most intimately. We know what we have to do to get our bread here. We know exactly what we have to do and how we have to dress for other people to pat us on the back and say that we're nice people. We know EXACTLY what songs we have to write and sing in order to get on Top of the Pops.

We know it because we've lived this all our lives.

The reason that we are not doing it, especially us here in this room, that we are not acting on this information is because we have a knowledge about the real universe, know what a travesty the concentration camp is and we don't really want any part of it.

We don't want to engage with it because we believe it is in essence a DENIAL OF THE REAL UNIVERSE.

But that's up to you, because it is insane and because of that it actually doesn't make any difference, because the construct concentration camp is insane, and *it doesn't make any difference what you do here*.

The universe is looking at this human concentration camp and sighing sadly, and it is looking forward to people evolving out of that and not doing THAT any more.

But whilst they are looking at this, they are also completely aware that the insane actions taking place inside there cannot be held against the inmates.

The true laws of order don't exist here.

Now, the entire universe is ruled by love, this is correct; but the concentration camp is not ruled by love but instead, it is ruled by fear.

That is our first and most profound difference between the real universe and this human made bubble of madness.

So when you see weird shit like wars and killings on the television and you ask yourself, how is this possible? – well, this is how it works.

It has nothing to do with God, literally and practically nothing AT ALL.

This is people going insane in the prison of their own making.

The real universe is ruled by love and by FLOW, and it is magical in nature; the concentration camp is ruled by fear.

It is not ruled by pain as such, because if you push up the fear enough, you can get someone who might get to be a hundred years old without ever really experiencing physical pain beyond a tap with the hammer on the thumb when they are hanging up a picture of their grandchildren on the wall but they still live in fear their entire lives.

This is just FEAR, not fear OF anything at all; and it is fear that holds this insane prison together.

I don't know who started this, who did this, who made this; I'm not interested in that, but I'm more interested in making a hole in the barbed wire and say to some people, "Hey, let's go! Let's go out into the REAL universe because everything you ever wanted is THERE."

Happiness, joy, feeling at ease, feeling as though you belong, making a proper contribution, living a real life – all of that is OUTSIDE of that concentration camp, always is, always has been.

Those who run the concentration camp will post their border guards, and they don't like us sneaking out.

So, I'm going to put the word FEAR into our diagram.

Fear is not just the barrier to magic.

I have this essences book called, For You, A Star. It has all this stuff in it – dominion, freedom, joy, love, all sorts of things. Delight, *pleasure*.

Fear is the one single enemy to all of them. You know this, but I don't know if you really appreciate as yet how far reaching this is, and what it does.

So I am going to bring you briefly up to date with the single most important piece of research Nicola and I did in the course of the last year, and which has brought about the most tremendous threshold shift.

A Matter Of Fear

Now, we tend to think of fear as something we have once in a while, every so often, it comes like an attack and goes away again.

So you're sitting there and you think you're not afraid, and I sneak up and go, "Booo!" and then you are frightened.

But this isn't how it works and it's a mistaken idea because it presumes that you are at Zero Fear Point before I came along.

We are not.

Our concentration camp, the Hard, has a BASE LEVEL of fear that is actually HIGHER than what a zebra experiences when a lion comes running towards it, and there is scientific evidence for this.

A resting human being in a relaxed state has MORE adrenalin in their system ALREADY than a zebra has AFTER it had its adrenalin shock when the lion came around the corner.

We all of us live constantly in a base level state of fear. Now we can ask, "How the hell is that possible?"

HOW is that possible?

Let's make an imaginary scale with a point of zero fear and if we move back a little bit, Western humans are on a minus 500 units of fear level when they are resting and when they are asleep.

When they are *asleep.*

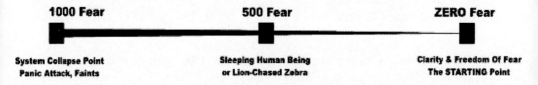

This is why it gets ever worse, the older you get; this is why people can't produce HGH in sleep any more because these kinds of stress levels are like trying to sleep with a pack of hungry lions right outside your bedroom window.

You just don't sleep properly, every little sound can wake you up, it's an alert sleep state.

If they are THAT afraid WHILST THEY ARE STILL ASLEEP, how afraid are they going to be when they get up in the morning, go downstairs and see a letter on the doormat that's possibly printed in red, or has "Law Courts" written on it?

Now, we are talking TERROR – instant TERROR.

So you put on the radio and they say we are expecting any minute now hundreds of planes flying into buildings anywhere, or envelopes with deadly poisons delivered to Polegate, East Sussex – actually, into YOUR very house!

Now this wouldn't be a problem in and of itself apart from the fact that it destroys your immune system, destroys any chance of ever being happy or relaxed, because all the good emotions are of course on the other side of that zero fear point, right?

- **Any hope of intimacy, any hope of connectedness, any hope of anything <u>is on the other side, past the zero fear barrier</u>.**

But what it also does is that fear makes people incredibly STUPID.

The more stressed you are, the more stupid you become.

It's a form of tunnel thinking that occurs, you see less and less, this is the structure of panic and panic attacks, when people see something that stresses them out, let's say you got a summons to a Law Court – that letter is all there is, that letter is the entire reality, all there is and all there could ever be.

Stress focus, tunnel vision.

They are not thinking about the fact they are married to a lawyer. That they've got seventeen million pounds in the bank. That they are very pretty and will do well in prison.

They are not contemplating any of these things, all there is is that one letter.

Imagine someone who is in that state and is making decisions based on not the whole story but stress controlled on just one little aspect of the bigger picture that they can't see any longer because they're too stressed is the leader of a world nation with their hand on an atom bomb device?

Or is making decisions as to what the police is to prosecute, or what wars should be fought against whom?

What kinds of decisions are being made under stress?

STUPID decisions, of course.

And it is this what has left us with stupid religions. With stupid rules. More fear inducing nonsense all around us. With stupid laws. With stupid divisions between man and woman, black and white, children, grown ups and old people and how useless they are. Stupid traffic systems in East Sussex – my God, you should see what they've done in Tesco's car park. You cannot believe it was possible that anyone could ever have thought that it was possible to get cars in and out like that?

It's unbelievable, and I've always asked myself that question, how can people be so god-damned stupid and so short sighted?

This is how. They are so stressed and the more stressed they are, the worse the decisions they make, become.

Unfortunately, our stressed out muppety leaders have worked out that if you make people *even more afraid*, they become very easy to lead, because you can put that tunnel vision of fear like a beam of light on anything at all, let's say, on the Jews.

Everything that's wrong with you, EVERYTHING, the fact that you can't feed your family, that no-one loves you, that you have no self esteem, that's the Jews fault. Lock on target. They're everywhere, they have a great conspiracy, they have weapons trained everywhere, if you just destroyed that one thing, if you get rid of that Law Courts letter, your life will be fine again ... ready, steady, go!

This is happening all the time.

At the moment in the UK we've got a witch hunt on for smokers. Not the first, not the last, I remember one from twenty years ago where the target was dogs. Every newspaper was full of attacks by Rottweilers on innocent children, and everyone was going blind because the dog faeces were up to our knees ...

It's bullshit.

It was bullshit then, it is bullshit now, it will always be bullshit.

These witch hunts are being whipped up by society leaders is usually because there's something going on just there, outside that stress circle, and if they weren't so stress focussed and panic struck, because people are actually very, very intelligent.

They have more neurons in their heads than stars in the visible sky. They have lifetime's experiences with liars and idiots. The only way you get people on mass to act stupid is by making them afraid.

So they are making them more and more afraid of everything. And then we get stupidness, real stupidness.

God loves one religion, but not another.

Yeah, right ...

Can't eat fish on Fridays ...

Ookaaayy ...

We MUST have a man come with a stick and knock three times on the door of the English parliament, and then slam the door in his face or else it's not a proper session.

Rrrright ... oookay ... that will help us with our current problems of unemployment, won't it ...

So now, this fear thing, you can see how it works globally and how amazingly it turns nice human beings into killers and concentration camp guards.

How it turns intelligent people into stupid raging lunatics that any wolf would raise an eyebrow at, and say, "What the hell is wrong with that species?" Sharks would shudder at the behaviour of very stupid, very stressed out people going absolutely berserk on mass. They would, and you know that.

That may be so on a global level and horrendously impactful societally, but I don't actually care. What I am much more interested in is that **if we are afraid, we cannot actually do any clean magic.**

We are not thinking straight, and a lovely example is evoking a demon.

The poor idiots didn't know that they weren't evoking them, they were MAKING THEM. You make a thought form, like Alister Crowley in his three day ritual, to evoke some demon that some person with a good sense of humour wrote about in some book in the 12th century.

So this original writer had a bit of a Project Sanctuary experience with a thing with tentacles, probably because his father used to beat him brutally, so he wrote this thing in this book, and now Alister comes, 800 years later, and he wants to evoke this demon.

But of course, it isn't THAT demon at all, it's a demon Alister makes himself in that three day ritual in giving it all these attributes and all these energies, and pouring it all into this one contained thought form that becomes then denser and denser, and there comes this point in space and time when our friend Alister can't tell the difference between his own hallucination any more and a lump of wood.

This is simple human functional pathology.

Now he's completely convinced he's made a demon, and if there are other people in the room, in such a trance, they will see it too; and now, we have a demon which really exists – no, Alister, it didn't exist at all until you made it, but now it does and it's still around somewhere out there.

But just imagine you were making a demon, and you were slightly off in your energy because fear makes you unstable and stupid, and it makes you doubt yourself so you are no longer sure what is what, AND it cuts the feedback mechanisms from your body and from your energy system.

This can make people so stupid that they can't tell any more which mushroom is actually poisonous simply by looking at the thing and feeling it in their body, getting a kinaesthetic kick that makes them flinch back, "Whoa, I'm not eating THAT!"

So if you get people to that point, then you get ONE GUY to write a book on mushroom, give them all a book on mushrooms instead, and ...

Bye, bye, intelligence.

Bye, bye, magic.

We are now in the hands of those WHO WRITE THE BOOKS.

Fear Creates Poisons

Not a good state of being, is it.

No. Because now, you've actually lost the one thing that could get you out of your prison cell, which is the direct connection to the Creative Order, which is why I made you do that exercise with the plants outside.

That's you and FERN.

That's you and a tree.

No book in between that tells you how you should feel, what you should think or what is good or evil about it.

So, and knowing and this is so, how are we going to use this to our advantage?

We have to get rid of our fears.

All of them.

I mentioned earlier imagine what happens to a person, not even a magician, a person who has been told that oil gives you heart attacks, that it makes you fat, that it means that no-one will ever love you again, as they are putting some oil into a sauce pan because they want to fry themselves an egg, because if they didn't, it would all get stuck horribly to the bottom of the pan and you wouldn't get it out and it would be disgusting and a mess.

We have created an autogenic poison.

We have created an autogenic poison for the energy system.

That is a really good example of how the fear of something **makes that something poisonous.**

Everywhere else in the universe oil is the greatest gift ever.

You ask a polar bear what he makes out of the rich oil reserves of the seals he eats, or what would happen to him if he didn't get access to that.

You ask a seal baby what the oil in its mothers milk can do for it.

Ask an arthritic what fish oils can do for their joints. They can actually answer.

Oil isn't poisonous but we make it so by OUR FEAR OF IT.

Aha!

We make things poisonous by our fear of them.

The fear itself turns something that isn't poisonous into a poison, and that goes for mostly everything, not just for oil.

That goes for love, and all the other good things we find in the really real world. The only way you can stop people from looking for all this good stuff is by making them so afraid, they won't even try.

Hands up who's afraid of love?

Honestly?

Ok.

Hands up who's afraid of magic?

Real magic?

REAL magic?

Ok, fair enough.

We have some honest people amongst us, either that or they don't really know what love is, or magic, because *they should be afraid*.

Really ...

So what we need to do is we have to treat our fears of things, and most importantly, of things that we don't even know we are afraid of them but they are causing this endless background noise of fear that stops people from sleeping deeply and producing HGH whilst they sleep.

Which is prematurely ending their incarnations here, and is keeping them in a constant state of low performance.

You can eat as many vegetables as you want, you can exercise as heartily as you want and you can sing "Om!" as much as you want, with that base level of fear, health cannot be had.

Intelligence cannot be had, and clear thought cannot occur, and that's a fact.

That goes as much as for anyone sitting here today as it does for a seemingly young and healthy executive of 25, full of the joys of spring, who plays squash, he's terrified the same as the rest of us that anyone might find out his girlfriend isn't as pretty as he said she was.

It is OVERWHELMING what we are afraid of, how many things trigger our fears, how it is constantly, constantly re-affirmed in everything we do and everything we say.

So I've got one little magic spell – just one! – which is quite nice and is quite simple.

NLPers and affirmation guys might not like this, but as you are holding your bottle of oil in your hand and before you put it into the saucepan, you look at it and you say, "I'm not afraid of you any more."

You could go on to say something else if you wanted to, such as, "Actually, I love you. You WILL BE GOOD FOR ME."

Next, the egg.

What's in the egg? Will it increase your cholesterol?

Isn't there something evil in eggs so you have to boil them to death or else you get some sort of disease?

Can we fry this egg without that fear in the back of our minds that we're about to risk killing yourself, your loved ones and everyone else you held dear?

Are you starting to wish you'd made scrambled egg instead?

But not on white bread, because that's BAD for you ... Brown bread, but even that's not good enough, it's processed. Actually, we should be eating handfuls of grains instead and no eggs at all, because the Buddhists say that you can't eat any living thing ...

Christ!

As the Germans say, "Guten Appetit!"

Enjoy your meal!

Let the health of this wondrous meal flow through you ...

Can you imagine just for one moment, your day, from the moment you get up?

What do you think?

Brushing your teeth, putting on some skin cream whilst being dubious about its results, or whether you really should or not ...

Soap, water ...

Is your tap water safe? Didn't I read in the newspaper that it is over-chlorinated, that it contains all sorts of evil, and might it not be far too dangerous to brush our teeth with that?

Perhaps we should get bottled water – but what's in the bottled water? Can you be sure?

Oh ...

Just let these things come to the surface for a day, sit back fold your arms and just have a look what kind of lives we're leading here.

And as you're putting the clingfilm around your cheese, there's a part of you in the back of your mind which goes, "Oooh, there's some sort of wandering component that goes from the clingfilm to the cheese and that is carcigenous ..."

It is actually AMAZING that any of us are even still alive with all of that going on – it's true!

Every little thing we do is just totally covered in this evil slime of fear inducing misery, and it would be really nice if we could remove that – but not yet, you don't have to.

I don't want you to change your lives right away.

What I would suggest is that you just sit back and WATCH THAT GO BY.

Sit back, fold your arms and watch yourself being terrified – of your mail, of your children, of your loved ones, of your carpets, of your washing powder, of your bread, of your nail polish, of your hair products, of your cellulite, of your own face in the mirror – whatever!

Just get an idea of just how much of that there is, and be amazed that you have managed to cope so well under these circumstances as you have.

If you really wonder why you've made such shit-stupid decisions in your life, well, that is why.

THAT

IS

WHY.

People who are afraid can't make good decisions, they can't see the bigger picture. They just do any old weird thing to make the pain stop, get a break, they make really stupid decisions – and we have, haven't we?

Some of us are more willing to admit this and quite enjoy it in hindsight, and wonder how it could have been possible that we ever thought THAT could have been a good idea, it's quite funny when you get to that point.

But, fear HAS GOT TO GO.

With fear gone, clarity increases immensely, and so does SENSITIVITY.

Now we've been told that we should not be too sensitive, "because it'll just hurt more".

Now really!

What is that?!

It'll HURT more if you're more sensitive?!

What about sex?

I once saw a man, strapped to a wooden cross, being beaten by four grown men and women with REAL leather whips, with knots at the ends, until he was a bleeding mess, "not feeling anything".

He was rather disappointed; he undid himself from the thing and dragged home sadly, "I didn't feel ANYTHING ..."

This is true! I have witnessed this!

You have to be sensitive to read and navigate the patterns of reality.

In order to do ANYTHING with your life, you have to be EXTREMELY SENSITIVE, and I'm going to give you just one example where sensitivity is of the essence.

And I don't want you to think of sex, or how great that feels, all the wonderful spiritual aspects of it, or how it makes your toes tingle, and how it seeps up into your ...

I just want you to FOCUS.

Magic & Luck

What do you ladies and gentlemen make of "luck"?

Would you like some?

Now let's first of all strip away the nonsense that luck is winning the lottery. That's not luck, that's some sort of stupid muppet dance.

My son Steve calls it a "muppet mash".

Winning the lottery isn't luck, it's actually nothing, really.

How is that going to make you any happier?

It's so not, is it.

It is one of these illusions that you hold up to the inmates of the concentration camp, as a *fake target to dream towards*, so that they don't think of leaving it.

The illusion says that if you win the lottery, people will start to love you and respect you, that you can buy health, youth and good feelings and that you don't have to be afraid any more, right?

That's the lie; of course, it isn't what REALLY happens when people win the lottery. They just have an extra couple of million quid and other than that, they're the same miserable son of a bitch they always were.

It is a fact; look at the history of lottery winners. This doesn't give you anything of REAL value, because everything that is of real value is of course OUTSIDE of Muppetville, outside the concentration camp.

Including luck.

- **Real luck is when you are in the right time and in the right place, in order to make something happen that will happen IF you are in the right time and place, but nowhere else.**

Shall I say that again, slowly?

Luck is – say you want to find a boyfriend, or a girlfriend. Let me be more global. Let me say that you want to meet a particular person who will significantly enhance your incarnation with their input.

Now, people who are lucky will know exactly where to go to stand and be, and that person will come by.

It will be a particular time and a space – let's say, 7.15pm on the street corner opposite Lloyd's bank.

Not on that side, but on this side.

On that date, at that time you just have to be there and stand there and wait, and the person will literally fall into your arms.

You know they will; you stand there, put yourself into the right position, wait for it, and – there it goes. It happens.

That is luck.

Right time, right place, matching your desired outcome?

Remember magic?

Getting EXACTLY what you have designed to have happen? Your will manifest? Not just some random weirdness?

Now, if I desire a rose quartz crystal, and someone throws a lump of jet at my head, that isn't luck, that's a random weirdness.

Or someone comes over and hands me a bunny rabbit – that's not how it works, that's random noise.

Luck is when I want a rose quartz, and I get EXACTLY that.

It's expected, it's desired, it's designed – and in order to know where you should be, WHEN you should be in order to get that which you desired, you NEED TO BE SENSITIVE.

Sensitive to WHAT, you may ask?

Have you ever heard of astrology?

We have this big golden thing in the sky called the sun, and this has energy fields and then these other planets hopping about, and the laylines of the earth. You've got universal weather, to which the sun reacts by making solar flares, and all of that you might call an energetic environment, an energetic landscape.

This is a fluent landscape where all the components are shifting and interactive; it's not like saying, there's a tree over there, and we'll meet by that tree.

The energetic landscape is made of elements that move and shift, and they move in time.

Today, the lucky spot is near Lloyd's bank; tomorrow, it will be on the other side of town in the park by the big tree.

You need to be able to discern when and where these things occur in order to make use of them, and have your luck happen.

Many people use this. They don't just randomly plan trainings, for example.

It might not be random where or when it is held, and it might have nothing to do with how much the venue costs.

It might not even be question of it having to be a weekend, it could be any day if there are other considerations at work.

If you want to do luck "the hard way", this would be walking into a place in Las Vegas with a lot of slot machine.

And somewhere in that room, there is a "luck convergence" spot for you. Right vibration, right machine, right time of day. It's a big room. It might not be 100% but it will pay out three times what you've put in.

And that's the one to pick.

Which one is it?

In order to pick out the right one, you have to be sensitive to this.

The Auspicious Time Exercise

What I'm going to do is to ask you to do is to think of something you would like to do; a special little project, nothing too dramatic, just a project that you have had in mind for quite some time and we are looking for an auspicious time to be starting this.

Does everyone have such a project in mind?

Maybe painting the garage, or starting the Atkins diet, whatever comes to mind.

Or starting to write a book perhaps. Starting a new business. Deciding on a new colour for your kitchen. Anything you would like to do.

Have a little moment to be clear that this is the project you want to be working on.

Where do you feel that in your body?

Let the energy flow and keep the energy of the project, and the idea of the project, steady until it flows quite nicely and there are no major blockages or reversals to the idea remaining.

> If you need to do some
>
> Softening and flowing, please
>
> By all means do,
>
> So that at least
>
> The experience
>
> Of this one project
>
> Is nice,
>
> And clean,
>
> And smooth,
>
> Before we start
>
> To consider
>
> When the right

Or…

> "Auspicious" time
>
> Would be
>
> To do that
>
> In actuality.

I am going to ask you first of all, for a time of year, just globally.

Is it spring, summer, autumn or winter that would suit the beginning of this project the most?

I would then just like to ask you simply for a time of day – morning, afternoon, evening, night, anytime including the peak of night, dawn perhaps, sunset.

You will feel the compatible energy from the project asking you and guiding you to something that matches that quite nicely.

And now, just for fun, I'm going to bring in the muppety concept of the days.

I'm going to let the days go by you and you pick the one where you get a strong sense of yes, or which is the most compatible with your project's desires and energies.

Monday

Tuesday

Wednesday

Thursday

Friday

Saturday

Sunday

Ok, now you can open your eyes and you've learned at least the day and time of day within a three month range – and I could have done the year's month as well but I couldn't be bothered.

And did you find a nice match between the energy of your project and an auspicious time?

<Audience agrees>

Yes. And was it also quite clear which one it wouldn't be, couldn't be, some sort of weird feeling that it just could NOT be that – Friday? In the middle of the night? You're kidding me! That is the WORST time in the World!

Why?

"Ahm ... I don't know, it just FEELS really bad ..."

And that's the right answer to this exactly.

Sensitivity to feedback on such things is the key.

This is nothing other than Art Solutions again.

You do not need to consult complicated star charts or look at at the phases of the moon to find the right time to do that love spell you always wanted so badly to do.

This time, you are going to get it it RIGHT.

This method of simply matching the energy of your desire to another thing works for all matters of rituals as well.

Custom Rituals

Now then, what's a ritual?

A ritual is something natural that we do step by step so that the poor old lonely conscious mind can keep up.

A ritual is something like EFT, that the conscious mind can remember in a moment of disturbance if it is practised enough, like counting rosary beads.

Rituals are designed to alleviate fear.

Now you can ask people who switch light switches on and off a hundred times what that is, and that is of course also a ritual.

The structure of the ritual stops the conscious mind from freaking out.

So that is why magic, and religion, and teaching, and sex has ritual aspects – people use rituals for these things.

But we are going to re-define this ritual meaning into that it is **a sequence of events IN ORDER TO GET SOME THING DONE.**

A ritual is simply a step-by-step sequence of events that leads to a desired outcome.

We had a nice example of a mini ritual in the Art Solutions question: "What of this food should I eat right now to make me feel happier, fuller, more full of energy?"

This question opens up a sequence of events.

Next, you get an answer, if you are sensitive enough to pick it up, or if your marps have been given enough freedom to just go and get the thing, and you take it and you eat it and that whole behaviour has been completed.

That's the original, essential meaning of any ritual – you want to do something, and the ritual is the path to get it done.

Now you get incredibly complicated rituals over the ages, especially if many people chime in and add their bit. It might have started out with one red candle and "Please bring my lover to me now."

You let thirty or forty witches at it, and you have half a dozen candles, seven different kinds of flowers, nine scarves, cinnamon, brandy, dancing, singing, horns, knives, cups, salt and all kinds of outrageous nonsense – and the ritual has become A MESS.

This is why so many rituals that are currently being run seem so messy and pointless.

Because they are.

This thing we just did, where we took a project, have its energy flow clear so that it flows nicely and we don't have any reversals, no fear, and THINK CLEARLY about it; and when we localised it in time, a season of the year, a day, a time of day, in order to do that on that day, gives us our require outcome.

You don't do rituals for ritual's sake, you do rituals for a required outcome.

A lot of people forget this – a lot of church rituals go on and people seem to have forgotten what the point of it ever was, but they all DO have a point – if they don't have a point, then don't do the ritual, in other words.

What we are going to do is that we are going to CUSTOM DESIGN our own rituals.

And that's as easy as pie.

It really is.

Do you remember your project that you wanted to get started?

Would you like to have a go at designing a ritual to support this in the secrecy of your own mind?

Yes?

Ok.

Let me ask you to simply tune back into your original project.

Let the energy of the project be with you and flow through you, so that you have something there to compare it to, because you make that comparison of the energy of the project and some other existing things which also have their energy and their vibration.

- **What we are looking for is something that is at the very least compatible, if not the very best match you can possibly make.**

I am simply going to ask you to look around for a mineral, a gemstone perhaps. They are great favourites amongst people doing or trying to do magic, because they are lovely. They are very clean, very clear, no matter what the muppets say about what they've done to them; the crystal's own energy overwhelms it, within a few hours anyway.

So what it might it be?

Might it be a clear quartz, or a rose quartz?

A red obsidian or green agate?

Might it be turquoise or emerald, or ruby?

Either which way, find a mineral energy source to support your project, something that matches, near enough or perfectly.

And now we have our gemstone, let's also have a silk scarf, just for the fact that they hold colour so nicely. That will be our symbol for the colour of our project.

Which colour should our project be associated with?

White?

Yellow?

Orange?

Red?

Pink?

Violet?

Blue?

Green?

Turquoise?

Black?

Silver?

Gold?

Just pick the nearest match.

Very nice.

And that will do us for now.

Did you find a gemstone and a colour?

<*Audience assents*>

Very good.

Now what can we do in a ritual with that colour?

We can wear clothing of that colour, we can design a symbol in that colour, we can have a candle of that colour. These things are all designed to bring that reality of that thoughtform, that outcome we desire, cleanly, and that is the word here, CLEANLY, into existence.

Simply, the more aligned the energies of a thing are, the more powerful it becomes.

This is also known as Zen, or as congruency, integrity – that's when all things are matching, when they are working together on a similar level.

Now that basic sensitivity of matching energies of one thing to another FOR A SPECIFIC OUTCOME that's really magic.

That is what magic is – and simple it is, too.

Let's have a flower to go with your project!

What flower do you have?

Passion Fruit Flower? Amazing! They're quite alien, and cool.

Pansies? Nice, like little butterflies.

A rose? Cool.

Sunflower? Ah, the queen of daisy like flowers!

Well, look, this is all very nice and friendly, is it not?

It's easy.

It's not heavy, is it.

It isn't full of "whoooooo ... for your ritual ... three black candles ... and a small shard of obsidian .... whoooo ...."

It's only like that when you're freaking out with fear and panic and you think you're going to go to hell because you're not supposed to do it, and you shouldn't even be wanting what you wanted in the first place, and it's all nasty and eventually, it's all going to go horribly wrong anyway.

That's when you end up with rituals like that.

Rituals like this, they're not like that.

They are so easy, so simple.

They are led by your outcome – it is the outcome that sets the ritual.

And we ask and simply get the answer.

Could it be any simpler?

I'm quite embarrassed.

Even with the big alchemical stuff, it still retains this simplicity. If you want to do some big astrological thing for the most important of reasons, it's still as simple as asking, "Does your project prefer Saturn? Jupiter? Pluto? Venus? Mars?"

Simple.

A map of your town – "Where should this meeting take place?"

I am going to meet someone – where should this meeting take place? There? No. There, there? No, no. There? Oh. Warmer. And – ah, right there.

I wonder what it is – street corner, hotel lobby, it doesn't matter.

To do that and to **FOLLOW THAT faithfully** is the key.

When you begin to do that, and follow that faithfully in actuality, that is when this whole process begins to kick into action.

It's no good sitting there and saying, "Well in principle, that's ok, but in practice, no."

If you do that, then nothing will happen. There can be no magic.

But I can guarantee you one thing: if you start trusting that a little bit, or even a lot – we are at a point now where we trust this so much, well, we wouldn't even be here, any of us, if we didn't.

I would not be standing here today in front of you if I didn't.

I have learned to trust this, because it is a better way of CALCULATING REALITY than when you are stressed out and you're trying to make a decision, and you just KNOW that you haven't got all the facts.

How could *anyone ever* consciously make a ritual?

You see people trying, though.

They have five magic books open, ten, and "Oh but in this one it says three red candles, and in this one it says only two, and in that one it says you should use cinnamon, and in that one ... oh, I better try and put it all together ... damn, I've forgotten to sprinkle the salt and I must ring the bell five times ..."

That's no magic!

That's just ... terribly, terribly SAD!

Put down those books, dear lady!

Take off all those crystals from around your neck!

Here, sit down.

There, have a cup of tea.

There, there now.

Ok ...

Let's put all this rubbish away and start from the beginning with what you need – which colour should it be?

It's so simple, I hang my head in shame.

That's how you make rituals.

It's how you make potions – again, it's embarrassing.

Do you remember the ivy potion for the back of my legs from earlier?

Now let's see.

How am I going to take this ivy potion?

How am I going to make it?

Do I go out and buy "essence of ivy" from the Bach flower remedies?

No.

Would I like the homeopathic ivy?

Absolutely not!

That's a strong physical NO response I had there, it shuddered right through my body. Whatever homeopathic ivy is, it has absolutely nothing to do with what went on between me and that ivy out there.

Would I like to put the ivy leaf in a glass of water for a while and then drink the water?

Yes.

That's as simple as that.

You list the various options you have for making any potion, put all the options side by side and simply go along with your feelers, with your internal dowsing rod, and just find out when it starts to twitch – that one!

For me, just the idea of ivy transferred into some water will do the trick, whereas the essence would do nothing and the homeopathic version was completely wrong.

Is this going to help you choose your remedies?

What do you think it does for you when you ask YOUR SELF rather than asking a book?

<Audience Member: It would empower you.>

Right. Empower is the right word for that. This is empowerment. As you use this more and more, what you are gaining is TRUST in YOUR SELF.

And money can't buy that.

This is not just about successful projects, making potions, getting demons to materialise in the Hard, but far more in you learning that you can trust your self, that there are things you can do for your self, and that you can get to know what is best for you.

This is the core reason why I couldn't recommend playing with these little rituals highly enough.

Now, I have got a job for you to do in the lunch break.

I want each one of you to design a small ritual for your project, something that you can easily do in your kitchen. I don't want anything that requires vast earth-moving machinery, a cast of thousands and stage lighting at this point. We'll do those later.

Keep it simple, keep it small and confined and so it helps your project, from the beginning to the end, and when you're done with it, it will help your project and it will considerably enhance the chances your project has of succeeding on this planet.

An Exercise In Movement

Before we go to lunch, I'd like us to do a little movement exercise.

Put your books away and rise lightly, and with pleasure!

You can shake your feet out, and then shake you autogenic feet out as well.

It's one of those instructions I love – I really don't know what people do with that neurologically, but it's always worth a smile.

Have a move and a wriggle.

Do you remember your symbol for feeling better from earlier?

Yes we won't be using this one, we'll make a brand new one for this exercise.

<*Audience Member: A different one?*>

Oh goodness, yes!

There's a universe full of them, never ending, for every purpose, each flavour, most delicious each one!

This time, we are going to do the symbol with the other marp, so it also gets a turn.

This time, I'm going to ask for a gift for your energy system.

And for mine!

An unexpected gift, a DELIGHTFUL surprise, and let that movement occur.

The movement is the energy, the symbol is just what keeps our conscious mind amused as we look at the pattern being drawn, but it is the movement itself that spreads out from your arm into your chest, and into your neck, because in fact you can't move your hand without subtly moving your entire body.

Your entire neurology can become engaged here for a moment and support that symbol, that movement –

Your toes can help as well,

And your spine,

And your hips,

All parts of you

Join in,

And let this movement

Be your gift,

And when it's flowing all happily and nicely, we're going to stop, clap our hands and say, "Thank you, marps!" and go to lunch.

Part 3

Custom Rituals (continued)

The Spirit Of The Thing

In this session I am going to start talking about the spirit of a thing, or the underlying energetic reality, and words, for example, symbols, and our lives in this dear concentration camp of ours, otherwise known as The Hard.

The Hard is outside of God's laws, or rather, it tries to be – it is an endless struggle that can't be won.

Our favourite metaphor is the fruit tree.

At some point, it was decided that we would be better off if the branches instead of reaching up towards the sun were to go sideways instead. To make it easier to pick the apples.

Generations upon generations of gardeners have tried to "train" this fruit tree with ties and bindings and cutting and chopping, but *the tree just never learns ...*

One day, the gardener gets sick, and his son is away on holiday, and what happens immediately?

Voom! Everything grows back up.

The insanity of Muppetville, or what people do and think they do, doesn't actually make *any lasting change in reality AT ALL*.

It can't.

And that's a wonderful thought.

Now, it's not much consolation for those who suffer in utter misery under its rules and regulations, of course.

People in starvation camps. Christmas is coming, and then there'll be the multitude who will launch themselves off of rooftops, or use up their remaining stored up supplies of Ritalin to put an end to their meaningless existences. Those who no longer have what it takes to put an end to their meaningless existences and so they go on nonetheless.

You can see those in their droves in the local supermarket at Christmas time; the sadness and the misery on mass can be quite overwhelming.

But on the bright side, don't worry about it.

Seriously, this has been a real problem for the religions across the ages.

Yes, there is suffering; yes, there is terrible pain, and yes, it's completely meaningless AND completely pointless.

You don't get ANY karmic brownie points for this.

Not for any of it, not for any of what goes on in our concentration camp bubble here. And no matter how horrendous the suffering, or how horrendous it becomes what we do to others or experience at the hands of others, it is STILL essentially meaningless – it doesn't count.

Only things from the real universe count – they count, because they are real.

I see it as my job to bring as much information from the real universe BACK into this bubble, to make a bridge so that a flow of energy begins back into this concentration camp.

The easiest way to do that is the concept we discussed earlier of INTEGRITY – of aligning symbols of all kinds back to their real meanings.

Symbols & Structural Integrity

At the German EmoTrance practitioner training last week, this lady said, "I'd love to let more love into my life, but that feeling of BURNING SHAME is just so unpleasant, I can't ..."

I said, "I don't know what kind of energy you're letting into your life there, but it ain't love."

Love does NOT produce a feeling of "burning shame", it really doesn't.

Even the most distraught of systems, real love, star love if you will, HEALS us – do not all our prophets tell us this?

That love heals, it doesn't hurt, it doesn't judge – there is no "healing crisis" with unconditional love, with REAL love.

So what happened there was that this lady was, at some time, treated with certain energies. She was exposed to certain energies which produce in any normal person that feeling of "burning shame" and pain – BUT she was TOLD that this energy was called "love".

Now and naturally she rejects love; who wouldn't? It is most sensible of her to reject that stuff she felt back then.

I had a T-Shirt with "Love Sucks" on it.

It doesn't suck.

But what happens is that our concentration camp has a special language all of its own.

- **And this language does not correspond to the real existing realities in the rest of the Universe.**

So here we have a thing called "love", an essence of love, an energy of love, just what Plato was talking about, an absolute existence of an energy form called love.

But that is NOT what people talk about when they talk of "love" inside the concentration camp.

When some guy has just beaten his wife again and says, "But I love her ..." is that the same as what the prophets talk of?

No.

If some woman screams insanely at her children and says, "I'm only doing this because I love you", is that love?

No.

But what happens is that these people grow up with a completely distorted reality which they think of as "love".

They will further make their very own custom made barriers against what they think is love, so that what could heal them, namely the real thing, can't come in and heal them.

- **So what we have in essence here is a basic INCONGRUENCY between the word, and the essential reality it is supposed to be describing.**

There was another lovely example.

We did the Rainbow Connection, where you take two ereas and link them up so that an information exchange can take place.

This lady absolutely refused to connect up two ereas, namely "love" and "force" because "nothing good can come of it".

I pointed out to her that love without force was a weasely, pathetic thing that had no power at all and wasn't worth having, and that force without love is some horrendous travesty that you might as well call rape.

This is a classic mislabelling problem.

Love is the greatest **force** in the Universe.

It is A FORCE.

It is POWERFUL.

It CREATES CHANGE.

It washes away all sorts of nonsense and debris – it is **forceful**.

It is the THE most FORCEFUL thing there is.

But this lady thought that force = rape, and love = some pink, meaningless, pointless thing like a Valentine's card or something.

And she acted upon this AS THOUGH IT WAS REALITY.

This is what in essence creates the concentration camp of Muppetville in the first place, that is how it comes into being.

Generations upon generations, the words, symbols diverge ever further from the REAL reality they are supposed to be describing; and it gets ever more bizarre, ever more illogical, as time goes on.

In Energy Magic what we do is to bring our words, colours, actions, behaviours, plans, goals BACK with the realities we find OUTSIDE, so that there is a congruency between the words and symbols we use, and the energy behind them.

What is currently being done is that they take the word chocolate, but instead of real chocolate, put a slimy piece of poison into a wrapper, with "Chocolate" written on it, and they sell that to children who HAVE NEVER TASTED REAL CHOCOLATE, and they think that slimy shit in there ACTUALLY IS chocolate.

This goes in all ways. You can get addicted to slimy shit, like Heroin for example. It doesn't do you any good at all, it doesn't help you with anything whatsoever.

This UTTER confusion between reality and symbol, including words, then creates madness, like the famous Coca Cola advertising slogan, "It's the REAL thing".

That doesn't make any sense to anyone at all, yet it sells millions and millions and millions of bottles of Coke – because people just cannot give up searching for love, magic, joy, fulfilment, all those real existing energies because they are programmed as creative order beings to always seek – pleasure.

I love that you cannot train that out of people, no matter how much you beat them, torture them, try to destroy them.

Even the last beaten up vegetable in a mental asylum will STILL have it in them somewhere along the line to try and find PLEASURE.

You can't stop it.

So our charlatans come along with all kinds of fake things, a candy here, you open it up and it's just worms – but people can't stop buying it.

And that's NOT because they are stupid.

It's because they're PROGRAMMED to want it, they KNOW that they NEED it, and it is RIGHT that they should want it.

That they should try with their last breath to get it.

So let us say we wanted to start and start to re-define some of these key words.

Here's one – love.

We defined it earlier – can there be any objection to seeking THIS?

Do we desire this?

More than desire this?

NEED this, with every fibre of our being?

Oh yes.

So when we do magic and we ask for "love", what is it we ask for?

A pretty boyfriend for the "tossing of the salad" ?

A new puppy?

Can you SEE how utterly essential it is in magic that you should be completely AWARE of what it is you're asking for? And to ask in the right way?

How about the concept of Beauty?

Now that has become such a travesty, you can hardly read the word anymore.

What is Beauty?

Britney Spears, right?

Ah, damn, she's a bit past the sell by date now. Ok, so let's say, Britney Spears how she was five years ago.

Is that beauty?

Nope.

Is the Taj Mahal beauty?

No!

It's made by a person, so how COULD it be?

Duh!

Beauty does however really exist as a concept in the real reality.

Compare the Taj Mahal to a sunset, and you know what I mean.

This is the kind of "beauty" that leaves you speechless, breathless, whether you are religious or not, on your knees and with tears in your eyes because you really don't know what to do with those energies anymore.

So if we are doing magic and we're doing "beauty", WHAT KIND OF BEAUTY should we be asking for?

Let's talk about wealth.

What is the meaning of wealth?

Big house, big car, 3 accountants, 12 lawyers.

A "landscaped garden" with a swan lake as the centre piece.

Is that wealth?

It's SOLD as wealth in the slimy stickers?

Is THAT what you want?

No.

Force, power – all these concepts are NOT what we were told they are, and the reason that many of us are in personal development and end up saying, "I don't know why I am self sabotaging myself, I don't seem to want wealth, love, beauty, power, joy ..."

Joy?

What's "joy"?

On a sunset terrace with a gigolo and a glass of red wine?

What is that?!

That's not even vaguely a pleasure – even if **you know how to do pleasure.**

Pleasure isn't something that just falls on your head like a 16 ton weight, but it's something you need to know how to have, like an orgasm.

It's something we do – to take pleasure in things.

So let's say we wanted to write an affirmation or a spell.

This is a nice example.

Focus On Structure, Not Effect

Why do you think energy self healing is so incredibly ineffective in most people?

I've figured it out.

When you bring a person into hospital, on a stretcher, and they're screaming, "Ouwh! Ouuuuwh! Aaaahrgh!!!" what are they thinking of?

Are they thinking of their INJURY or are they thinking of their PAIN?

Their pain – right.

So if you give them a choice whilst they are in pain, and we say, "Alright, now either we can repair what is causing this, and the other is just take the pain away, which one do you want?"

Of course, they'll say, "Take the pain away!"

No matter how enlightened we might claim to be, when we are in the first person position of being the client AND we are in a great deal of pain, when we do energy healing, we ask AUTOMATICALLY for pain relief and NOT for structural repair work of that which is causing the problem.

What happens when you ask for pain relief when there is a structural problem that is using the pain to get attention?

You can expend a lot of power and get NO results at all.

I'm sure you've tried it.

Raging toothache.

Soften and flow. Tap, tap, tap. Pray, pray, pray. Three laps round the Krishna statue in the garden.

And the pain's not going away, is it.

"Fuck this! Magic doesn't work. It isn't real. Oh, but I knew it ... Deep down I always knew I would be sooo disappointed ..."

The thing is with magic and all energy work, INTENTION really counts.

You can't lie here in the real Universe.

You can't lie, you can't pretend, and you can't be any better than you really are.

In Muppetville, you can go and see a plastic surgeon and plaster on a lot of paint and then you "look" as though you're healthy.

On the energy levels, it doesn't fool anybody. They see you for the Picture of Dorian Grey you truly are – haha!

For example, in self healing we must thereby ask for the injury to be healed, and NOT for the pain to be taken away, because your systems would resist that.

It is not holistic, cohesive or even logical to "just take the pain away".

I hate to state the obvious but my ex husband really did take out the bulb from the red oil warning light in our old Cortina. He did. It annoyed him. He reckoned that it was spurious, random and the car didn't really mean it.

When the engine ground to a horrible halt for the lack of oil one day, and nastily so at 40 mph, it came to our attention that it had not been spurious, or random, and to take the oil warning seriously next time.

Now let's bear in mind that this isn't a character defect but indeed a natural thing to want if you're in pain for the pain to stop.

But actually, for well being and for the future – and we are VERY interested in the future here, because there is sod all you can do about the past! – for the future it is ESSENTIAL that we take our focus away from healing any kinds of pains and to repairing the structural injuries instead.

So if you are given to praying, instead of "Please God make it stop!" the prayer should be, "Please God, repair the underlying injury!" because that WILL make the pain stop, and quite quickly too.

Energy healing is remarkably quick.

I'm sure you have all helped OTHERS experience very, very fast and dramatic shifts in well being – it's a bugger it doesn't work for yourself, isn't it?

That's because when you are helping another, you have the bigger picture. When you're the one who is in pain, you are INSIDE of the situation, you are stressed, you get stress stupid and you miss the point – obviously.

However, we can do better than that and remember in times of stress, that we need to be dealing with the problem and put our intention and energy on repairing the problem.

This gives us some very nice guidelines as to how to structure magic spells.

But before we do that, do we have anyone here who has an energetic injury they have tried to heal because it bugs them?

This does not necessarily have to be physical pain.

It could also come out as relationships pain, money pain, success pain, performance pain.

These are symptoms, are they not?

People who have, for example, money problems, and I'm sure there's no-one here who does, but those who do, outside those poor deluded few who have money problems, will have an array of symptoms.

They spend too much, for example, and don't get enough value in return. They will fail to save. They also fail to make the most of opportunities that present themselves, and generally speaking, they would be completely out of control with their finances. They probably won't want to look at them, get very stressed out about them, and the whole thing is just a mess and a chaos.

Now what these beginner magicians would do if they got a hold of a manual on magic, they would just ask for more money to alleviate the pain, right?

But that doesn't work.

That is like shouting for more morphine if in fact you have a bullet in your chest.

It doesn't help.

Your systems **know this** and so you can pray and pray and pray, and witch and magic and call in the angels, the demons, the saints – you are not going to get any move on it AT ALL.

Because money is not the problem!

More money WILL NOT alleviate the problem and your totality knows this!

Funnily enough, the more enlightened you become, the more aware you become, the more spiritual you become, the bigger this problem becomes – because you are becoming a better magician!

Now when a complete muppet stands there and says, "I want more money!" their energy system doesn't even hear that. Their physicality isn't even in the same room. They are in that strange space where you have Wall Street and competitions who has bigger cars, and their bodies are just not there.

They get their payback and their heart attacks 30, 40 years later.

But us lot, when we are talking about such things, we need not to be talking about taking the pain away, but instead about REPAIRING THE UNDERLYING STRUCTURAL PROBLEM.

Money Injury Exercise

Who would like some more money in the hard?

Hands up?

Ok, I think we shall do an exercise. A classic EmoTrance exercise.

What I want you to do is to feel your money problems for a while, and then back up from there, take the bigger picture and ask yourself, where is the most important injury? Often people have more than one, but we want to deal with the most important one located in your body.

The one that is driving all those many symptoms. The one that unless you repair that, we can chuck a lottery win at you and it is just going go through those same injury systems and it's completely pointless to give you any more money because you'll lose it just the same again.

I'd like you to do that as a pairs exercise, if you would.

Do it in the classic EmoTrance fashion.

Where do I have this injury in my body? If I knew, where was it? Where can I feel that pain when confronted with bills? Dreams where you think, ooh, if only I could afford that lovely healing clinic in the sky ... That pain, you know where that injury resides.

And this time, we're not going to be asking to take the pain away, because that's a waste of time, but we're going to repair that problem and heal that injury.

When that injury is healed, you will not be wasting money anymore. You will not be leaking money, and you will be able to handle it, not be in such confusion over it, and you should learn to like and love it, even, because it is no longer a problem to you.

Would that be useful to you, ladies and gentlemen?

Would you like to do that, with all your heart and soul?

Because there is still a part of us that is stuck in this concentration camp, and money is a key to power in this concentration camp.

Ah!

It may not be of God, it may not be of the real world, but a part of us is stuck in that place, and here we need to have these injuries revoked so that we can shape our incarnations to our own liking, and in keeping with our plans for this, our lives.

Does this make sense to you?

This ends the conflict between spiritual enlightenment and money.

Money does not buy you happiness, by a long shot, but large injuries in the energy system because of this foreign and bizarre energy which exists here is not going to help anybody either. It is going to give them endless stress, problems, headaches and trauma and it really does impact on their effectiveness down here.

So are you clear on what you are supposed to do?

Money injury, find it, heal it.

And I want you to do this really in depth, give your partner EVERYTHING you've got by the way of help and support.

I'm going to give you 20 minutes for this exercise, so really go for that, and make a REAL DIFFERENCE in THAT person's life, right here, today.

Go!

Life Raft On The Sea Of Details

The reason I wanted you to do this exercises was so that you have an experience, and an example of dealing with the cause of a problem, rather than the symptoms of it.

When we are stressed, the first thing we do is we get lost in a sea of details.

You can hear this when people ring up, or see it when they write an email without paragraph breaks, full stops, and commas. You know these big blocks of texts from stressed people that arrive in your inbox?

There are no paragraph breaks, no **breath is being taken in** between and there's this whole litany of, "And I was abused by my father and my mother beat me every day and my step brother was in the Mafia and my therapist was a Satanist and ..." so it goes on.

These are all details, all these details flowing in and they are very, very stressed.

When people think about their own problems, they are in that First Person overwhelmed stress position and with the money it is like, "Oh and I spend too much and I don't earn enough and my mother never earned enough either and I've never had an experience with being rich and I'm just not lucky with money and numbers frighten me and ..." on and on ...

Focussing on the underlying problem rather than that stress stream of symptoms makes it much easier to heal what has caused this.

Also for relationships: "My husband doesn't love me and my children hate me and at Christmas time I'm alone under the turkey and ..." on and on.

Heal that relationship problem, it's a lot easier, it's a lot quicker and it is also delightful because you get a lot of feedback of the magical variety, or what our poor concentration camp inhabitants *think of* as magic.

So they do this money injury repair thing and next thing there's a cheque in the mail from someone they haven't heard of in ten years.

How is that possible? How does that work?

It must be magic ...

What they all said about there being a sea of infinite abundance and prosperity of all kinds, whether this is relationships you want, joy, luck, prosperity, whatever, being OUT THERE, pressing in on us to get in, and all we have to do is to dig a little channel, through our own defences as it were, to start flowing in, through and out us, and bring us its splendours and riches – that's all true.

It's all completely true.

There are incredible amounts of money out there.

Incredible amounts of people who are looking for a place to put their love and their attention.

Everything you want is out there, and we stop ourselves from receiving it and that's a fact, a real base spiritual principle.

And now that you know that, and you know how to repair the problem, we can apply this to a great many things.

Whatever causes you mischief in your life, turn it around and repair the underlying injury, rather than staying with the multitudinous symptoms of it which can be confusing and frightening. That way we make some real progress towards the things we want to do.

And this brings me very neatly to the concept of directional affirmations and magic spells.

Directional Affirmations and Magic Spells

What is the difference between a magic spell, a wish and an EFT opening statement?

I'm so glad that I don't have to explain this in German, because in English, it is simply the last line:

As I will, so mote it be.

It is really interesting, isn't it?

An EFT opening statement would be, "I'm having terrible problems in my relationships" – tap, tap, tap.

Or it would be in Choice, "I have wonderful relationships."

But what it doesn't have at the end is, "AS I WILL SO MOTE IT BE".

Can you feel the difference?

As I will so mote it be.

There are some amongst us who aren't that familiar with spells and witchcraft.

There is this word, "mote" and the reason it is phrased like that is because in ordinary street English, we don't actually have a word like that, and in ordinary street German, the entire sentence doesn't exist!

Not even amongst the magic practitioners!

This is a sentence that states:

This is my will, so shall it be done.

However, they used the word "mote" not "done" because "done" is a bucket and a spade, and a concrete mixer – and that's not magic.

Let me be quite clear about this.

If you want a wall in your back garden, and you go to B&Q and buy the bricks, buy the instructions, buy the concrete, mix the concrete, lay the foundations, build it a brick a time, that is NOT magic.

That is doing it "the hard way".

Is that quite clear?

I have to make this clear because there are a lot of people who go round saying that first you do your magic spell and then you go out and buy the concrete and the wheelbarrow and the instructions.

Those people haven't gotten the hang of magic at all.

Building a wall by magic does NOT involve you and wheelbarrow.

The question remains whether we should be building walls by magic at all.

Or what magic is for.

I went to see Uri Geller and he is really fascinating.

But the amount of energy he expended to make a compass needle move by 2 degrees was quite frightening.

I thought he was going to burst a blood vessel.

Now you really could say that the wrong torque wrench is being employed for the wrong screwdriver, couldn't you.

Really!

Magic is not for building brick walls.

What it is for is **for creating shapes and patterns that become reality.**

To make the plans for the house and where it will be built BEFORE the brick layer arrives – THAT'S what magic is.

Magic writes the book before the artist has put his first hand to the first key. Then the gremlins come along and print the whole thing and distribute it, but it is quite an important and interesting distinction here.

Human Will & Reality Creation

So let's talk about this "will" business.

Can human will make any lasting change in the real universe?

Can the application of human will make any lasting changes in the structure of time and space?

No.

Anyone who believes this really needs to go see a psychiatrist, the old fashioned ones, with the electroshock therapy, to knock some sense into them.

They can create an ILLUSION of change, like forcing a fruit tree to grow sideways, but that's about it.

Give it a few millennia, and see what's left of that "amazing change" in the history of mankind, time space and the universe.

Have any of you seen pictures that the Hubble space telescope brought back?

Have you seen the pictures of the galaxies and every one consists of a million billion milky ways, and every milky way consists of million billion stars with their own planets and solar systems?

Do you really think anyone gives a toss whether McDonald's serves salads nor or not?

You think that is a contribution to the greater order of things, do you think that MATTERS?!

It matters only in this reality-confused, bizarre, encapsulated space I've called the concentration camp. I'm sure, some species refer to it as purgatory.

I'm sure of it.

We might all be here because we did something really, really BAD when we still had tentacles!

But that's fair enough in and of itself, isn't it.

- **So, what we can use our will for quite tremendously is for changes that relate to anything in the concentration camp.**

And if you think to what degree our actual lives consist of worrying about what other people think of us, how much money we have in the bank, whether our kitchen floor is clean – or not; what we think to ourselves before we fall asleep at night, I would say that even for those people sitting here, that is STILL 75% of their daily grind.

Muppetville rules still 75% of everything we do, AT LEAST and if not more so.

We live in it, don't we.

I drive along all enlightenedly in the Even Flow at 275 miles per hour, and I go past a speed camera and just watch what happens to me!

It's true, I can flow. I can drive my car quite safely that fast, I really can. But try and explain that in a court of law, or to a policeman.

There's a higher part of me I call Lord Ashtar, and I hand the steering wheel over to him, and the marps deal with the rest.

You know, many good people who were confused between what's in the concentration camp and what's in real reality, have gone round and said things like this in all earnestness and found themselves in prison cells, laughing stocks, and in real stocks even, having tomatoes thrown at them.

But we can avoid this by retaining a sense of reality.

Now, will works with those rules of Muppetville, and it allows us to write them *at will*.

At **will**.

Just to give you an example how it works.

There was this really disturbed bloke, didn't have much of an education, didn't have much of a sex life, and he created this bizarre thing that terminated in the Second World war.

His name was Adolf Hitler.

Now a great many people don't like him, but if you are interested in reality creation he is an interesting point in case.

You can take other people. Some carpenter from Nazareth, if you want.

The fact remains that Muppetville is and remains completely UP FOR GRABS.

There was this guy who went round and declared that you cannot accelerate a human being past 25 miles an hour or their internal organs will explode.

As I will, so mote it be.

People were having HYSTERICS when the trains went down the hills, they were having epileptic fits, tantrums and their internal organs near enough exploded!

Well the brakes failed and the train went down the hill and it went past 25 miles an hour – you'd be surprised.

There were Victorian ladies who would FAINT if they had an original idea or "thought too much".

Doctor Atkins has created this bizarre reality whereby you eat whole cows and buckets of lard, and you lose weight and your cholesterol goes down.

Well it's true – look!

Look, look how easy that is!

One of my favourite examples is, someone at some time invented this whole Father Christmas deal and now everyone is running around in circles, shopping, worrying, crying because their family isn't under the Christmas Tree ...

WHAT Christmas Tree??

WHERE did that come from???

<u>Somebody CREATED that.</u>

We can create these things!

And what do you need to create these things?

A little bit of no fear, a little bit of congruency, and just the knowledge that no-one will be able to tell the difference!

I'm going to tell you the snail story.

I'm sorry, but it's got to be done.

The Celtic House Warming Snail

One time, my sister-in-law moved house, and I forgot all about the house warming party.

My father-in-law came to pick me up and I had no house warming present. So I just grabbed a brass snail from the shelf on the way out.

When she came to get her house warming present from me, I gave it to her, looked her meaningfully in the eye and said that it is a Celtic house-warming tradition, to give people a snail, upon the moving of the house, because the snail carries the house on its own back, and is always happy in its own house, and it's never homeless, and thus it is the traditional ancient Celtic symbol of house-warming.

She nodded all through my speech, took the snail from me and I thought no more of it.

I thought it was neat, but it didn't really go beyond having overcome the problem that I'd completely forgotten to buy a plant or something.

Until about six years later, my mother moved to England, and we had a house warming party – and my sister-in-law turns up with a snail.

She hands it to my mother, winks at her meaningfully, pats her on the back and goes off to the buffet to get herself a glass of wine.

My mother, who was well brought up in Germany to be polite, whispered to me, "Is she completely insane?"

And I said to my mother, "No, actually, it's an ancient Celtic tradition. Because the snail carries its house on its back, ..." and my mother went, "Oooh ..." and took the snail and carried it off most happily.

Now that would have been good, and the end of that, if I hadn't been at a house warming party some years later – and this guy comes in with a damned snail!

Completely unrelated, completely different set of people, and I'm like, "Why are you bringing a snail?!" and he's says, "It's an ancient Celtic tradition, because snails carry their houses on their back! You fool! I'm astonished you don't know this!"

And it tracked back to some person to whom my sister-in-law had given a snail to in London, and they knew someone else, and they knew someone in Liverpool, and that person knew someone else, and that was the connection that brought that other snail into that house on that day.

You can take that as far as you like.

Snail Day.

That's where we celebrate that we're not homeless.

We give each other snail cards, and the children go from house to house, with shells on their back, dressed in green, and they do a little dance, and we give them dollar bills, because they are green like salad and snails eat salad, right?

It's completely logical, makes perfect sense and is COMPLETELY MADE UP, from the ground up.

Oh dear, oh dear.

Will you do me a favour, people?

When you get invited to a house warming party, will you take them a snail? Or a card with a snail?

See, the next thing that's going to happen is that someone who got a snail house warming card will do an archaeological dig, and they will find some sort of calcified snail, and they will go, "Aha! An original Celtic house warming snail!"

And then we have the timeline established, right back to the dawn of time, complete with exhibits in the national history museum – *as I will, so mote it be.*

Now, I'm sorry I did this, it was a complete accident at the time, and I didn't know what I was doing.

But it is an indication what you can do, and how easy it is.

And that it makes absolutely no difference to the greater order of the Universe whether inside of Muppetville, they dance around with snail shells on their backs or go on about some giant rabbit that paints its eggs.

What the HELL is that?

That is so unlikely!

Christmas crackers!

What IS that? This thing and you pull on it and a hat falls out – as a meaningful symbol of family togetherness?!

It's just incredible.

The world is completely up for grabs.

Who Do You Want To Be

The only real truth is OUTSIDE of Muppetville, everything inside is INSANE and you can do what you like in there.

No karmic debts, no nothing.

The problem is this, of course.

If you have got so far that you can see this, of what love and beauty really is, would you WANT to increase the suffering in Muppetville?

Can you, even?

Can you be evil?

"Oooh, I'm going to be really evil and hurt these people ..."

It's pointless – you can't hurt them.

Can you heal them?

What do you think?

I think we can. I wouldn't be here if I didn't think we could.

If I didn't think that we could IMMENSELY improve the conditions inside this concentration camp.

A bit of basic mental hygiene.

Basic, decent nutrition.

Not running around thinking that beauty is Britney Spears, age 16.

That's three things already we can make a good start with.

Most important is to know that whatever our lives are in the context of this bizarre construct, WE get to decide – WHAT do YOU want to be?

Do you want to be a pop star or a martyr? Do you want to be a granny? Do you want to push a shopping trolley down the streets and mutter insanely? Do you want to be all of these things in sequence?

What do you want to do?

WHO do you want to be?

Once you understand the principles of Energy Magic, you will know that this is not prescribed.

A long time ago, there was an illiterate peasant girl who ended up leading the armies of France.

If THAT is what you want to do, you can do that.

Not so long ago, there was some black guy in a prison somewhere who became the symbol of the freedom of black people in South Africa.

There was this old nun called Mother Theresa. She became a symbol of loving care for the less fortunate, and a HUGE inspiration for so many people.

WHO DO YOU WANT TO BE?

That is what "As I will, so mote it be" means.

It doesn't mean you get a cheque on the doormat, it is much, MUCH bigger than that.

You can choose who you want to be and what you want to do.

And don't give me the rules and regulations of Muppetville, because they are baloney.

There are ways and means around that once you know.

Have you heard it said that there is one law for the rich, and another for the poor?

This is true.

So, if you seriously wish to contravene the law, what do you need to do?

You have to become very, very rich – very good!

Now you're getting it.

Muppetville has its own rules and regulations, and you know what they are exactly, because you were born to them, you have experienced them and lived them every day of your life, and you know how they work.

So, who do you want to be, people?

Just for now – you don't have to settle this forever.

I thought that I would be a great dog trainer one day, and, actually, I was, a really great dog trainer. And then I thought, ok, I'm bored, let's be something else.

Have you ever thought of yourself as anything other than what you thought you wanted to be?

Are there things that you could never be?

Ah!

As I will, you mote it be.

Let's chunk it down a bit.

When you ask people, "Who do you want to be?" they usually wax lyrically and mystically, or they say, "When I was little, I wanted to be a train driver."

Now we come to a very interesting thing – wish fulfilment in this incarnation.

Wish Fulfilment To Unlock Incarnations

When Sandra was a little girl, she wanted to become a marine biologist because she thought this meant swimming in the open sea with the fish, like you saw on Jaques Cousteau.

She thought that this would be magical, and very, very desirable, and thought that the way to get to that was to become a marine biologist.

Which is good thinking, completely logical, and there is nothing wrong with that whatsoever.

Now, we are here, and our organising principle is PLEASURE.

Give her that, that little girl, let her have THAT.

It's not difficult, is it.

Even if you didn't have much money, you could still put a quick trip to the Mediterranean with a diving holiday on your credit card. With Easy Jet – 220 quid, that's not hard.

That's cheap to fulfil life long wishes, that are hanging around in our energy system and that IF THEY WERE FULFILLED, would allow us to let go of that and move into the NEW, and think of new and DIFFERENT things to do with this our life, no matter how much of it there may be remaining.

So the question of who you want to be can be addressed on many levels, but you should be ALL that you could be.

What I would like you to consider in the break – and make a little list! – is who YOU always wanted to be, who you thought you could never be, and know that you can fulfil that, because in this incarnation, as people and in this set up, we can do more or less whatever we want – if only we know that, and know to follow the conventions that run the real world, and the human made prison camp, respectively.

Not only can we do what we like, we can also do some good, WHILST having enormous amounts of fun.

Now, we have Sandra teaching classes.

We have Sandra teaching classes right now, and then we have another Sandra teaching classes AFTER swimming with the dolphins.

Is there a difference?

When do we have MORE Sandra?

When do her students get MORE Sandra?

More delicious Sandra?

She is already delicious, but what WE BRING TO THE PARTY is what counts, whether it is politics, accounting or lecturing, teaching or writing, what we bring to the party is OUR SELVES.

If what we bring is sparkling and bright, and brilliant, and that is completely in our hands, then therein lies a trifold benefit:

Of getting what you want;

Of having the time of your life;

AND having a chance of making a difference inside the prison camp.

So have a think about that, and come back with three things you want to be when we return.

Part 4

The Duty To Make Dreams Come True

Fasten your seatbelts ... for the last session, our soaring flight into many alternate realities which are right here and right now.

Right here, right now and nowhere else – they will never be anywhere else.

I spoke to some people in the break about their dreams and wishes they had when they were a child, and that was really quite interesting.

Oftentimes, I would hear variations on the topic of, "Oh but it's silly."

No.

It isn't.

Imagine for a moment you were a person who was completely in love with this other person.

Who always wanted to fly an airplane when they were a child.

But now they're 65 and have a stiff leg.

Would you not say to this person, "You can do that. You can go up with a flying teacher. You do NOT have to spend this incarnation not having experienced this."

Would you not encourage that person to make "that dream come true"?

The thing is that most people have such a horrendous backlog of wishes that never were fulfilled, and they waited for other people – Prince Charming, Mrs Perfect or the Mother Mary to come along and magically make their dreams come true.

And they waited.

And they are waiting STILL.

That's a fact.

It's one of those lies they have in the concentration camp, that you have to WAIT until SOMEONE ELSE comes along, and they give you permission or bring you this thing, dumps it in your lap or makes it happen for you.

That way, you can keep GENERATIONS waiting for something that never comes.

I had an intensely significant experience with this.

When I was a small child, my aunt died. She was 87 at the time and I happened to be there when she died. And her last words on this planet were, "I wish I had learned to play the violin."

WHAT IS THAT?

87 years old. Worked her guts out. Went to church. Tried to be a good person and live a good life according to the rules, did the best she could and beyond the best she could for her family, and what were her last words on her deathbed?

"I wish I'd learned to play the violin."

That's an extraordinary thing, is it not?

Now I said earlier that I want us to be smug on our death beds.

We will have learned to play the violin!

That doesn't mean to say we played it well.

That doesn't mean to say that people didn't run from the room screaming and said, "For the love of God, put that lethal weapon of mass destruction down!"

But I will NOT lie on MY deathbed and wish that I'd learned to play the violin.

That is totally HERE, that is totally **ACHIEVABLE**.

There are aspects of us that are so used to taking second best and not getting what they want, they've veritably given up; and these aspects of us that wanted to learn to play the violin, or to ride bareback on a horse, or to swim under the water like Jaques Cousteau, **those parts are the power to our magic.**

We need them on board.

We NEED them inspired.

We need them hopeful and delighted.

You HAVE to fulfil your own destinies, people.

And for that, we need a little bit of discipline.

Discipline

Now then, I used to think of discipline as this horrible thing.

But you see, someone had once again sold me this thing, marked "Tasty Sweetie", and you open it up, and it was cat shit.

Discipline is NOT doing something horrible, pointless, painful and flogging yourself against your will and want.

Discipline is the act of remembering what you want, and going for it.

Discipline is the application of will power in the pure sense of will power.

Discipline is when you decide that you want to learn how to fly an airplane, and the old muppet thing comes in, "Eeouwh, you're too old, and anyway, it's stupid and pointless and you should pay more attention to the stock market instead ..." to have that discipline to stand up for yourself and to say, "Oh fuck off! I WILL fly an airplane and that will make me into a better person.

"It will make me into a brighter, shinier person.

"It will say YES to who I am and give me what I need, and I may not even know what that is, but there is an energy about it and I promise you, you WILL get to fly an airplane."

That's discipline.

Discipline is when you get to write a poem, and you put your heart and soul in it, and you did it as best you could, and some critic comes along and says that it is rubbish, or stupid, or that you should not be writing at all, to have that discipline to stand up and say, "Get lost! These are my words, this is MY energy."

- **Discipline is the act of protecting your self from all that nonsense of Muppetville.**

Discipline is to make the complete dedication that you will remove fear from your life because it is the only thing that gets between us people and the creative order – and our own potential; and that if we are afraid, to have the mental discipline to take the steps necessary, to take the remedy, to draw the symbol, to stand up and say "I won't be afraid, I don't need this fear."

That is the core of true discipline – to be 100% on your side, to never forget that and to never waver.

It is a wonderful thing, because you see, the better you get at energy work, the more powerful and profound the thoughtforms and the energetic realities you are producing will become.

If you produce unfortunate and distorted thought forms, you will get cancer and give it to other people. You have heard of those healers who are always sick, right? Of "back firing magic"? The highest magicians in the land being these totally twisted, awful people that you would not touch with a bargepole?

Anyone here has ever seen a photograph of Alister Crowley?

Oh my God!

So much unhappiness! Pain! Suffering!

We have GOT to learn how to be careful in what we think, and how we think, and that is why we need our discipline.

The more we clear up our energy system, the more we step into who and what we are, the more sensitive we become, and the more effective we become in our magic, aka writing our own lives, the more important it is to think the right things.

Our poor little muppets, poor little poppets that they are, God forgive them, they are standing there with their oil bottle and they are thinking, "This is going to kill me, this is going to give me a heart attack, this is going to give me multiple sclerosis."

And because they're not really connected to their totalities, and their unconscious mind isn't really listening (it's off on the other side of the room with the pixies) nothing much is happening.

But when WE do that, we endanger ourselves, **because the greater our connection with the totality becomes, the greater our magic becomes, and the more important it becomes that <u>we think the right things.</u>**

Makes sense, doesn't it.

So for us, it is extremely important to stop whining.

We can't afford this anymore.

We can't go round every weekend somewhere saying, "Eeeouwh, my life is sooo baaad, and ooooh, I was so badly treated as a child, and waaaa ..." because we are calling these energies, calling these realities BACK into the room every time we do that.

These things may be true, and they may have happened, but we do NOT want these things in our present future.

In fact, the calling back of these old problems and the thinking about these old problems is what keeps them in the here and now.

So, in order to help us out with our mental discipline, we have some children's tools, namely prayers, spells and affirmations.

Magic Affirmations

Let's start with the affirmations because they are really quite straightforward.

Who dislikes affirmations intensely?

Ah, yes. That's alright because many people do.

Affirmations are totally pointless when the words that are being spoken and THE ENERGIES BEHIND THE WORDS don't match.

We discussed this earlier.

Someone stands in front of a mirror and goes in a feeble voice, "Grrr ... grrrr .. I'm a tiger ..."

Or, whilst crying miserably, "I'm a beloved child of the Universe ..."

Now come on people, we have all done affirmations like that, haven't we.

We were all miserable and depressed and whined tearfully, "I'm really happy ..." and it didn't work, did it.

Well and it wouldn't have, would it.

And it's understandable that we were a bit disappointed with the old affirmations and we decided that wasn't a good way forward, and indeed, for someone like that, it isn't a good way forward.

It's just a bizarre reminder of all the good things you can't have and you will never have.

So, from that place, they're really not very good.

However, there is a way in which affirmations can assist US at this point in our unfoldments.

Let's go back to my bottle of oil.

What is going to be better for us in the long run?

If we pour the oil and say, "This is going to kill us," or if we say, "This oil is life giving?"

Just the most basic neurosomatic, psychosomatic effect?

Fact is that it is immaterial if current science decrees that this oil is dangerous – we don't know anyway, do we. They are constantly changing their minds about what's good for you and what isn't. I love the idea of classifying McDonald's as "junk food".

Think about it.

We have baps made out of decent grain and good flour, right?

We have meat, from reasonably healthy cows, as far as that goes, but no worse than anything else you can buy in any supermarket. We have salad. We have tomato ketchup made with fine tomatoes that the creator gave us. We have a McDonald's hamburger.

We give this to any person in a starvation camp and what do they do?

They are going to shout, "Hallelujah!" and eat this thing – with greatest joy.

There is nothing wrong with a McDonald's hamburger.

It's FOOD, for God's sake!

People put all this STUFF on it – "Oh, this is going to make me fat, this is going to kill me, this is the enemy within!"

Well right it BECOMES the enemy within if you eat it with that attitude, and these enemy component structures ooze into every part of your cellular and energy system ...

Let's try and be sensible here.

We are going to use affirmations not so much in the first stage to create reality, but to STOP our selves from HURTING our selves some more.

Please!

We are going to use this to replace the thoughts we were used to having had, and which were so negative, and so deeply non-beneficial to our energy systems and our lives with OTHER thoughts.

Forget about "truth".

What do we know about "truth"?

It isn't worth the paper it isn't written on.

One person says this person is beautiful, another person says they're ugly.

I once sent an article to two editors and one came back with "It's the greatest article I ever read! This will save the world!" and the other with, "This is so disgusting, I would not want to insult our readers with this nonsense."

But that's Muppetville for you. "Truth" is one of those concepts that doesn't exist there, only "opinions". **Truth exists outside**.

So when we stand in front in front of a mirror, and this is a thing with affirmations, right at the beginning I said *we have to ACT AS A TOTALITY SYSTEM.*

The body has to act, the energy system has to act. The mind has to act, the energy mind has to act – all together and all at the same time if we want to make magic.

If you want to do these wonderful things they do in Zen – put a blindfold on, bow and arrow, target is five hundred yards away and smack! in the middle.

Me driving down a winding road at 225 miles an hour in perfect safety. That's magic, isn't it. And to do that, we have to be in the same place, at the same time.

And so in order to make affirmations work, we must learn to do them at the right time – and in the right place.

That's very simple, but they never tell you that about affirmations.

Would you like to have more luscious, glorious hair, anybody?

Yes?

So when would be a good time to make an affirmation to that effect?

When the sun is Leo?

No ... but ...

When you are in the process of brushing your hair!

Of course!

When you are brushing your hair, THAT is the time to affirm the shininess and strength of your hair – *and not at any other time*.

That is the ONLY time this is appropriate, because you are right there, with your hair, involved in the act of doing it.

If we want to make affirmations about strong teeth, when do we make those?

That's right, when we are brushing our teeth.

We're getting the principle here!

If we want a new, better car, when do we make affirmations about a better car?

When we are engaged in the act of driving.

Aha!

Now isn't that a different kind of magic?

A lady came over and asked me what I made of the habit of casting magic circles for rituals, and I laughed.

That idea was clearly devised by a fearful lapsed Catholic.

I don't want my magic to stay in a circle!

I want it to ripple and flow, to be a part of my life – of course!

In this way, we are bringing magic into every aspect of our lives.

Isn't that an interesting concept?

When will you make affirmations about how good an author you are?

Just before you start to write :-)

Of course.

Affirmations about being able to sleep profoundly, restfully, producing masses of HGH?

Before you go to sleep.

Of course.

What this does is to give your conscious mind something proactive to do.

When people have panic attacks and chaotic and miserable lives, their conscious minds are all over the place, because of the fear, obviously.

They are CONSTANTLY producing further disturbing and frightening thought forms.

This is going on CONSTANTLY.

And as we're looking then back at these thought forms, we freak out.

And the more we freak out, the more disturbing thought forms we produce.

Now you can't live life like that, never mind make magic, never mind make a contribution to your society, or alleviate the conditions in the concentration camp, can you.

No. Really, you can't.

So we really need to use some of these ancient tools wholeheartedly and correctly.

Look in the mirror.

What would be a good affirmation there?

I'm beautiful?

Yes, that's fair enough.

But then, you will HAVE to have the discipline to put a full stop to all the old thoughts of "Oh no I'm not because I don't look like Britney Spears when she was 16 and still fresh and peachy with those small little dew drops on her perfect skin ..."

There comes the discipline.

Now, people, are YOU willing to stand up against your selves for your selves?

Are you? Yes?

Are you willing to give this a jolly good old go?

Are you willing to understand that if you're thinking crazy thoughts you should do a round of EmoTrance or EFT or Heart Healing or take a bath? When you are having one of those moments, "Oh but I'm nothing special and it's all just an illusion and I'm meant to become maggot fodder and there's nothing beyond ..." to just realise that you've just slipped off into some adrenalin induced weirdness and you best not think anything for a while?

Yes?

Ok, very nice.

Crocodiles VS Golden Horses

This is a metaphor for Muppetvillian criticism.

The poor inmates of the concentration camp are used to defining THEIR reality by the comments others make ABOUT THEM.

They will decide as to whether they are any good at maths or not by some washed up, alcoholic idiot who doesn't even like his own species putting a bad mark under their maths paper in the 3rd grade.

You are TOLD that you are bad at maths, so there we are.

You are TOLD that you don't look like Britney Spears and that means you're ugly and you accept that.

See now, look.

What we are trying to do here is to **MAKE AN INCARNATION**.

This is not about going home, doing the same old rubbish and then lying on your deathbed and wishing you'd played the violin.

This is about making an incarnation for yourself, one person at a time, that counts for something, that was worth having, that was worth being here for and suffering the usual inequities we suffer whilst we're here.

This is what that is about.

Do you have the will to such an incarnation?

Desire?

Hope, even?

Yes?

Alright, so if you have the will to such an incarnation, then what we can't be doing with is crocodiles.

Let me explain.

Our incarnation is a cart, or possibly a beautiful wagon.

You can either acquire Golden Horses, or Crocodiles.

Now Golden Horses are all those things which bring their energy to help lift you in the right direction; Crocodiles are things that snap at you so that nothing can happen.

Let me give you a practical and personal example.

Whether I have a good voice and whether or not I am a good public speaker is neither here nor there.

Somebody said to me that they really liked the HypnoDreams, it was just a shame about me speaking, and whether Ananga could produce some without me.

Now that's what I would call a Crocodile.

HOW is it going to assist me in my growth as a public speaker if someone suggests that it is best for all concerned if I never speak at all?

How can I get BETTER at it with that attitude?

How does that help me, in general, even to come out of my house in the morning and say, "Hello, Mr Postman"?

It really doesn't, does it.

That's clearly a Crocodile.

That's like being told you're too young or too old, or to stupid or too thick, or too fat or too English, or too German or whatever.

It's a Crocodile.

It doesn't assist us but worse, there is NOTHING that is learnable from contemplating it. There is nothing that can be learned from it, it doesn't assist us and it is a terrible way of keeping people from what they want to DO.

Now there's a lovely swamp, 180 miles from here, where we can catapult such Crocodiles, and they will land happily and safely there.

So, I got a feedback form the other day about the HypnoDreams, where this lovely gentleman went on about my deep, rich, velvet alien voice.

Aaah ...

That's a Golden Horse.

I get told that, I try harder. I try to get better. I try to improve my diction.

And thus, my incarnational cart towards being a good public speaker with a nice, resonant fine voice is then well on its way, is it not.

Do I get big headed by doing this?

No.

Does it mean that either is right or wrong?

Aha – no, it doesn't.

In essence and in law, they are EQUALLY MEANINGLESS – but I'm going to use the one to further my purposes, and I'm going to catapult the other one out.

That's an example of taking charge of your incarnation.

I want to be a good public speaker when I grow up, and for me to have that be so, I really can't be doing with "Shut up and never speak at all."

You have got to go through your own areas of thought and eliminate the crocodiles.

And I really don't care WHO said it, and I don't care just how romantic the moment was, or how "true it may have rang".

Whether my voice is rich and velvety or not – compare it to natural realities. Does a nightingale sit in the corner and squawks, "Oh my voice is so rich and velvety, and I sound so romantic?"

Of course it doesn't!

There is no reality to ANY of it!

There is no pat on the back.

There is just the question of what you want to DO with this incarnation, and use what we've got here in our concentration camp to help us be the best we can be.

To enable us to do what we want to do.

Whatever that may be.

Is this a good way of dealing with "criticism"?

Indeed it is.

But it further avoids that special trap where everyone starts to tell me how wonderful I am, and I start to BELIEVE it.

Because you literally and practically can not take control of the Crocodiles, without understanding immediately and at the same time that the Golden Horses are of course, of that very same nature.

They are means to an end.

Some thing that you can use proactively and consciously to help us along.

That is the same for the words that we use, the candles that we light, namely to align ALL the energies available to us behind our selves so that we can go forward.

So, isn't that a nice thing?

Are we going to go out now and get some things done?

Some of these are going to be things which should have been done many years ago but weren't done, but they NEED TO BE DONE to unleash our incarnations.

Poor old Aunt Annie STOPPED when she was 6 years old and DIDN'T learn to play that violin, and nothing else then happened in that entire incarnation.

Wow.

Now this is dramatic, of course, but do you have such things in your incarnation?

Just imagine a 70% - 80% supercharge into your goal setting systems.

Wouldn't that be worth having?

Yes?

Good. Most excellent.

Freedom Spells & Totality Goals

A nice form of affirmation for EmoTrance practitioners are the Freedom Spells.

These are tools for this interim stage where you still believe you have a lot of this, that and the other, and the Freedom Spell is basically a structure which says,

"All of my ...

I now let you go,

Soften and flow,

Soften and flow."

Now they're good fun, because once you get started, you just can't stop.

You start out with, All of my heartache, I now let you go, soften and flow, soften and flow," and "All of my misery, I now let you go, soften and flow, soften and flow," and "All of my pain, I now let you go, soften and flow, soften and flow" and "All of my shame ..." and it just goes on, and on, and on, the first time you do that.

And it's a huge relief, as well as jolly good fun.

The more of these things you make an intention of not wanting to have anything to do with them anymore, this old CRAP which is weighing us down unnecessarily, where this is getting really funny is when you use the Golden Horse/Crocodile mindset and get to, "All of my achievements, I now let you go ..." and, "All of my triumphs, I now let you go ..."

That goes to Guiding Stars, so we get to have some new ones, some DIFFERENT ones, some exciting ones.

"All of my dreams, I now let you go – soften and flow, soften and flow!"

Most people have the problem that they dream the wrong dreams.

What we need are TOTALITY DREAMS.

You have to find some dreams that your whole person can agree upon – your body, your mind, your energy mind, your energy system, and even your soul.

And bearing in mind that what your soul is after, is possibly NOT a big house on the hill. Your soul might NOT be after you healing and helping and teaching other people for the rest of your life.

Your soul might be wanting you to learn to play the violin.

Aha!

So we need to make these totality goals at some point – an interesting point.

Can you now begin to see how I can stand here and say, "Once you've got a totality goal, you can put everything you've got behind that?"

Discipline, affirmations, every tool in the book – and do you think we then have reality creation?

Damn right you do!

And beyond mere reality creation – real incarnational creation, beyond just one thing to MANY things.

We can never know now what would have come AFTER that violin, can we.

It's a shocking thought.

My aunt was an extraordinary woman, and she really was. I mention her a lot because she made a deep impression on me. I don't know how much she could have done, for how many people, for her self, for the Universe at large if she had gone for the violin, and lived a real life, instead of having this half-misery existence of just doing her duty.

Heartbreaking. It is heart breaking.

And we can do better than that.

Because we follow the pleasure principle, for which the Creative Order designed us.

Thank God.

Energy Dancing

Now, we've been sitting here for quite a long time, have we not?

Well, you have been sitting.

I have been standing and walking about.

What I would like us to do is a mini party, if you will, not together, although we are together, but more of a mini party inside of your self.

Would you like that?

Have a little get together with the conscious mind, energy mind, physicality, all of that at the same time?

Would you enjoy that, do you think?

Do you think it might help with energy flow, and INFORMATION FLOW even if you will?

And would you like a little more Freedom?

Yes?

So what we have for you is the dance track from the end of Freedom, and for those of you who haven't heard that, there is a lady who is very keen on Freedom on that dance track.

What I will do is to have a little instructional tour as to a form of exercise that you might like to undertake by yourselves when you get home at any time you feel like that, or you need it.

It's an advanced neurological cross-wiring, while we're at it, and it is a little bit of hypnotic magic as well, but I think many aspects of you will enjoy this.

So if you'd like to put your writing materials away, lay down your shields and safely store your swords and your guns under your tables, yes, the knives as well, rise to your feet, or to your autogenic feet, as the case may be[1], and find yourself some space so you have room.

My voice in this venue is surround sound ...

---

[1] A live participant of this training had no feet, and another could not stand up because of physical injury.

So let us start to do some energy dancing.
Let's turn it up a bit so we can hear that beat ...
<*Music Track – Dance Track from HD3, Freedom, starts*>

>
> You don't have to start dancing
>
> Right away,
>
> You can just sway
>
> For now.
>
> Take a deep breath.
>
> And there may be some parts
>
> Of you today,
>
> After all that sitting,
>
> And working, and thinking,
>
> Who are not quite as comfortable
>
> As the rest of your body.
>
> And I was thinking,
>
> That on this occasion,
>
> Perhaps your toes can start
>
> To help out that part of you,
>
> By wriggling a little,
>
> Easing those parts of your body,
>
> Of your physicality,
>
> Of your energy system,
>
> Which may just be

A little bit stiff, or a little bit tense,
And in need of
Refreshing and
Awakening.

Perhaps your calves
And your knees
Might like to help as well,
They might like to make
Small movements,
That pulse through your
Neurology.

Your hips might like
To join in a little bit of
Soft movement,
Specially designed
To loosen your spine
And did you know
That little tail
You have
At the end of your spine,
It can move
And it can wriggle?

And all those parts
Of the spine
That are just above the hips,
Give them some movement
And let them assist
In this overall flow.

And I want you to notice
How this is already
Starting to loosen up
Some energy
And that is
Starting to flow.

Perhaps your hands
Might like to join in.

Every single finger
Helps to loosen
Blockages
And constraints
And constrictions ...
Your shoulders,
Your neck,
Your ribs might like
To have a go

And flex and flow
And everything
Wants it to be so
And we will get
Everything into movement,
Even things that lay
Asleep and dormant
For so many years,
Every part is called
To the party,
Every part
Every part of you
Every aspect of you
Everything in flow
In free flow.

Do you want freedom?

The tiny muscles around your eyes,
Locked jaws unfolding,
Everything joining in the flow,
Slow and sensuously,
Let the energy free flow
All through your body,
And have it feel great,
Have it feel marvellous,

> I wonder if finger nails can move,
>
> Ears can wriggle,
>
> Every one of your hair
>
> Becoming alive, electric,
>
> All over your body,
>
> At that,
>
> Wherever it may be.
>
> Ok, now we slow down
>
> A little bit and focus,
>
> On the energy system dancing
>
> Now, at the same time,
>
> And in the same way,
>
> As all the rest of us.

Breathe ...

Thank you very much!
How was that? Wasn't that great?

<Audience claps & cheers loudly>

Now here's something I'd like us all to do, and that is to have a round of applause, cheering and shouting your own name, cheering your self.

Yeah – all right!

How does that feel?

Isn't that wonderful?

How long did that take us?

Five minutes?

After the end of this long day, how do you feel now?

Loose? Alert? Vibrant? Prickly? Warmer?

Right!

And it's really quite simple.

Well done, may I say!

The nice thing about this is, when you are asking bits of you to join in the parade, that usually are never thought of. Your toes having anything to do with an energy blockage in your neck? You don't normally think that way.

But see, the marps are not just the hands, your toes have marps too, and the back of your neck – the body is a total body marp, really.

And if you ask your body to HELP YOU WITH YOUR OWN BODY, it's quite extraordinary – it's so nice!

When you notice that your neck is getting stiff, ask one leg, "What can you do to make that better?"

What it also does is it bridges those artificial divides we have set up in our autogenic mind and autogenic body, and it is a wonderful form of totality exercise.

Five minutes a day of this is guaranteed to be better for you and your incarnation than five mindless hours on a treadmill.

I promise you that with everything I have, for your long term spiritual, mental and physical welfare.

And it is rather pleasant!

For those of you who don't do much exercise, do you feel like you want to do this again some time?

Yeah?

And let that feeling just come over you, when you hear something on the radio or even just in your head, so that you just get up and have a little dance – your energy body, your mind, your body, all in the same time and in the same place.

So this is a first experience of what it feels like when we do something all together, and whatever magic you do, should FEEL THIS WAY.

Aha!

It's a guideline, a guideline towards states of being that get a lot better with practise, but are easy to do, even for total beginners, and have IMMEDIATE benefits for you.

Loving Yourself

Now the last thing I would like us to discuss is the question of loving themselves.

And if anyone wants to start loving themselves right away, they can do so. It's alright, we won't tell and this is just an audio recording ...

How many times have you heard it said that you have to love your self?

That you have to love your self first before anyone else can love you?

How many times have you "tried" to love yourself, and failed miserably?

Possibly because you had one too many beers ... no, just kidding. That wasn't the kind of loving your self I meant – or was it?

I don't know ...

But I had a bit of a revelation on the topic.

I understood something and I want to share this with you because it is really quite important.

Loving your self is a side effect of something.

There is something that comes before that.

And what comes before that is BEING IN LOVE with your self.

Do you all know the difference between "loving" and "being in love"?

What is it like when you are "in love" with another person?

REALLY in love?

What is that like?

It's rapturous, somebody said.

What a wonderful word.

Now then.

Do we have anybody here who is already – and constantly – RAPTUROUSLY IN LOVE with themselves?

Much sniggering and eye rolling is ensuing here!

I'll tell you something funny.

Muppetville is structurally set up so that you CAN'T be in love with your self.

Because you'd have to be a lesbian – if you were a woman.

Because you'd have to LOVE A WOMAN.

But that's not "the one", is it.

Because the "one" for a woman is a man.

And for a man it's supposed to be a woman.

The "one" who'll make it all alright, who'll make you immortal, sing you to the heights of sexual pleasures, who "completes" you and makes you a perfect whole?

Would you look for a same sex partner if you were heterosexual?

No, of course not. It's a big basic taboo.

Sure, you can "love your self".

You can pat yourself on the head, buy yourself a Valentine's card, but massively IN LOVE with yourself?

Ah! It's an interesting concept that you're not supposed to love someone like that who's the same sex as you, not be "in love" with them, anyway.

That's a first hurdle to really being "in love" with your self, and don't kid yourself, that's a huge hurdle.

We are so entrained to look for the other sex, cause that's where you get "love" from, and all those things you've heard about, so it just doesn't occur to us to look at our own mirror image.

But there's another thing.

Who's ever looked in the mirror and felt rather disappointed?

Do you know why that is?

Who's ever looked at a photograph of themselves and felt rather horrified?

Do you know why that is?

It's because they don't capture the beauty of who you really are.

<To audience member> Can I have you for a moment, please? Come here to me, sweet child ...

<Lady joins Silvia on the stage>

Ok, now look at her, but look at her, really.

Open the other pairs of eyes as well.

Get the feelers out and have a look at her.

Isn't she lovely?

Interesting?

Are you telling me that a flat mirror image could EVER even begin to give you an impression of who that really is?

Do you know that SHE HAS NEVER SEEN HERSELF?

All she has ever seen of herself are TRAVESTY REPRESENTATIONS, in mirrors, on photographs.

She doesn't actually know what she looks like AT ALL.

She has NO IDEA.

Isn't that amazing.

How old are you, may I ask?

Lady: 50.

Wow. Fifty years on this planet and she probably has all sorts of ideas of what she looks like or what's wrong with her, but she has actually NEVER EVEN SEEN HER SELF.

All she's seen is evil cartoons, and the mirror really isn't any better than that.

Does the mirror show you your beating heart?

No.

Does it show your energy system?

Does it show your lungs or the blood that flows through your veins?

Does it show your muscles?

No.

It isn't even a simplification of reality, it is NO REALITY AT ALL.

A photograph or a mirror or a painting doesn't show you any reality at all.

THIS is the ONLY reality of this lady.

The real thing.

This is the real thing.

And it is amazing! The real thing.

And she is just fascinating – the way she moves, and smiles, and does all those things.

You could spend a LIFETIME looking at this lady and never, ever get bored – but we don't know that about our selves!

We can SEE that about her because WE can see her, feel her, sense her, be in her presence, and enjoy her on all those many levels – but of course, a photograph doesn't give you anything like that.

So you look in a mirror, and OF COURSE it's going to be disappointing!

You might as well look into a Picasso painting, for what good it does.

It doesn't tell you who you are, and so unless you stop looking in mirrors and thinking that's who you are, it is going to be very difficult if not impossible to start falling in love with our selves.

Now we were all looking at this lady for only a short period of time, but are we not all already a little bit in love with her now?

<Audience concurs>

We are, aren't we.

Well how could you not be?

Let's have another person.

Let's look at this one here.

Same thing, isn't it.

Isn't she completely amazing?

With the hair and the skin which is now flushing lightly, and that delightful smile? Isn't she absolutely wonderful? And she doesn't know that either because all she's ever seen of herself were photographs and mirrors and she looked at those and went, "Urgh!"

Of course you would! Because they don't show you who you really are.

When you look at anyone at all like that, really look at them, it is virtually impossible to not find them completely riveting and lovable.

So.

Are you willing to accept that what you see in the mirror is not the truth, not the whole truth, so help you God?

<Audience concurs>

Are you willing to remember the next time you look into a mirror that what you're seeing there is God knows what, but it is NOT WHO YOU REALLY ARE?

<Audience concurs>

You are so much more than that!

By thinking that what you see on celluloid screens or in the cinema or in photo albums – it's not even ONLY an over-simplification, **it's just WRONG.** Of course no-one could love that and no-one asks you to.

But what I ask you to do today is to fall in love with your REAL self.

With your INTENSE potential.

With your sweet little quirks that you have acquired by chance, or misfortune, accident or misadventure.

You throw the crocodiles out and you learn to think of your self as this

PRECIOUS,

WONDERFUL,

EXTRAORDINARY

creature that you can be whole heartedly in love with, and not until you do you come home to yourselves.

This is not about loving at all, this is about BEING IN LOVE – furiously IN LOVE – with your self.

Will you give this your best shot?

Kick out the crocodiles, look at your incarnation and say, "Right, if I was furiously in love with this lady, what would I do for her, how would I help her out?"

"If I loved this man UNCONDITIONALLY, so much so that it makes me cry just to think about it, and I wanted to help him out in this life, what would I do for him?"

And you know what happens when you start to think like that?

You get to do the things for you that you have been waiting for other people to do for you.

And it isn't second best this time.

It is not only NOT second best, it is FREEDOM, because no-one can take it from you then.

If a big publisher comes along and says, "We're going to publish your book, we love you ..." Right ... and then they can go and take that away again, can't they.

Now if you love this person so much, you would give them your finances. You'd say, "I believe in you. I believe that if people got to read your words, they would love it. Here you go. I will raise a mortgage on my house and I will give it to you – here, take it."

Isn't that *something*?

And that way, it's real freedom. It is freedom from societal structures, freedom from having to lie and beg and contort yourself into some thing that you are not, and at the end of the day, only an un-contorted human being can bring the glory of God into the concentration camp.

We don't need any more lies, do we.

We don't need any more people who are good at lying or convincing.

We need some REAL truth.

REAL love, REAL beauty.

REAL power.

REAL honesty.

REAL joy.

REAL wonderment.

REAL MAGIC.

Are you up for that?

We can make this happen.

We have a beginning set of tools that if you work with these for your self and in your own way, you WILL discover your own ways to make it real and to make it right, and that's the only way – for the truth is a pathless land, and it cannot be reached by any religion, any organised society, any tour bus.

It's one person for themselves.

One person, one life.

One incarnation.

One relationship to God, The Universe and the All-There-Is.

And that is you – and me, and I think the best way to end this training today is for us to stand up one more time and to make a little pledge here:

I believe in the power of God.

I believe in the state of love,

And most of all,

I believe in me.

Right!

And one more cheer, one more applause, cheering YOUR OWN NAME, to set YOU up for a new way, for this incarnation that is YOUR incarnation, your life, on the future that is YOUR future, here and now!

<*Everybody cheers and claps*>

Thank you very much, ladies and gentlemen!

You have been an absolute pleasure being with.

I wish you a wonderful journey home and thank you very much for being here today!

ADDENDUM 1

In this Addendum, I have collected a number of prime examples of how one may use "Energy Magic" most practically in every day life.

The principle of Energy Magic, let us remember, is to:

Reconnect the invisible worlds and properties
back to visible, noticeable objects and occurrences so that
THEY ARE ALIGNED TOWARDS THE SAME END.

This is the same for making thought and behaviour congruent with movement and experiences of the physical body, as it is for speaking or writing words that have a UNITY OF FLOW in their underlying energetic structure.

It is a key skill which allows us to do all sorts of things – finding sequences of musical notes that evoke certain feelings and sensations, or even create a healing EVENT in our totalities; creating works of art, making decisions about our lives and how we structure them, and in the end, it effects every single aspect of how we conduct ourselves.

As all and everything we see, do, experience, deal with, think about, worry about and dream about ALL have these hard and invisible components, and as the rift between the worlds of what you can put in a wheel barrow and that which you sense with your other receptors has become so truly enormous in the last 100,000 years of human "civilisation", there isn't a single place, time, space event to do with humans that would not benefit from running energy diagnostics on what is happening, and CHANGING this in the name of congruency, efficiency and love of God!

What that means for us here is that there is just NO WAY I could even begin to give you an idea of the sheer width, breadth and depth of Energy Magic possibilities, applications, techniques and events.

All I can do is to give you some examples of "Energy Magic in Action", just some of the many, many things we have used the underlying ideas to make something new and useful, or to take something existing and aligning it better, making it more honest, more congruent and more workable.

These papers and articles are the tip of the iceberg, in every sense of the word. Restrictions in a physical book like this, and in the fact that at some time one must make a decision as to what to include, and what not to include, as well as deadlines to produce a finalised version are responsible for these articles being here, instead of the other (100s) of techniques and applications.

You can find these already existing ones, and the ones which are constantly, and I mean CONSTANTLY, being added by myself and others who understand the principles of Energy Magic, on the World Wide Web.

Please check in with once in a while, and please do NOT leave this book, thinking that "this is it".

It isn't. It is a snapshot in time – 2003 to 2004 to be specific! – and what was fun THEN, interesting THEN.

EmoTrance and Energy Magic are MASSIVE in their concept and of course, evolution and development is their first and prime directive.

I therefore truly apologise to readers 25 years from now for the limited selection here in this addendum, but with so much material, and so many possibilities, it was simply the best I could do.

So now, to the first of our Energy Magic patterns – a truly beautiful application, Project Energy, which in and of itself deserves far more than a full trilogy as it is just so useful, and user-friendly.

Project Energy

Welcome To Project Energy!

This is a truly exciting application of energy work and one I have personally enjoyed immensely.

No longer about remedial clearing up of the old, this is a confident step into a very different world, a very different way of doing something practical in the real world at that which at the same time becomes not just a step stone for your development – but a gift to you, a very real help in every sense of the word.

It gets better still!

Not only is this a bright and joyful magic, a million light years removed from all and every kind of dour or spooky metaphysics you may have ever encountered before, a magic that makes you sparkle and dance in all ways, but it is also the most wonderful process of learning and discovery for you and about you.

What we are going to do here is to literally create a special custom made project which you will bring to the world.

Something that is uniquely your own, something that has never been and could never be before YOU came to think it up and then take it right through all the layers and the levels into physical reality.

This project will for a change not sap your energy, but in the contrary, create a surplus of energy for you – and this energy will come in the form of money, of new learnings, of love, excitement and delight, in the form of gratitude and true admiration and acclaim from your customers.

It will move smoothly through its developmental stages and most importantly of all, it will have a truly sparkling identity of its own and HELP YOU every step of the way to make the right decisions, keep on track and draw all kinds of right and helpful energies to itself and to you in the process.

Sounds good?

Yes – that's because it is good!

It's actually better than you might conceive of at this point and before experiencing what this is, what it does and how it works.

Most of all, it is really really fascinating and it is FUN.

Projects without work, without procrastination, without irritation, without hesitation – Even Flow in other words and a chance to do something truly unique to human beings really, really well.

Are you ready?

Then by all means, let's stop talking and let's start doing some REAL magic!

Your Idea

So, you have a project.

A vision.

An idea.

Would it be valuable to you that instead of waiting and finding out if it will work, how it might unfold and experiencing what the problems will be in real terms, we could actually straighten all that out before we have even begun?

What would any project be like, feel like, that was entirely congruent, entirely beloved and entirely smooth in all ways to you and for you, that flowed with the ease of a sparkling brook, joyfully rushing towards the ocean, always downhill, always helped along by the sheer force of gravity, finding its natural path of the very least resistance and with the outcome being as certain as the rising of the day itself?

Well of course I cannot know about you, but to me that sounds pretty amazing.

And it is true, with hindsight I have already experienced something like this once in a while – a project that seems to have an impetus of its own, that comes into being so easily, so readily, joyfully even. It just appears, sometimes out of nowhere so it seems, and everything aligns – it even seems that the universe itself is smiling upon it as it receives help and support from everywhere and everyone and it so EASY.

But, if you are anything like me, it certainly isn't always like that. Not even most of the time.

Most of the time, projects SEEM attractive at the start but then they are beset by problems, by doubts, by details in which, it said, the devil himself lurks to trip you up.

The project that once seemed so sweet and such a good idea becomes ever paler as the original idea gets buried under a mountain of grinding annoyances – you know the kind, things are going wrong, telephone numbers misspelled, advertising deadlines missed by half an hour, important people's contacts, hastily scribbled on a piece of scrap paper and put "somewhere safe" irretrievably lost, machinery breaking down, outside events interfering ...

You know what I mean.

At some point you give up and think, oh dear oh dear, that was obviously not meant to be.

And if you're anything like me, at this point you sit down and shake your head and ask yourself, "Well if wasn't meant to be, then why on Earth did I put myself through all that? Why did it seem like such a good idea at the beginning? What HAPPENED?!"

The Dissonance Factor

The way I see it these days is that there was somewhere a dissonance between you and the project in theory or practice; a small dissonance for sure but for a long haul, even a tiny dissonance can make all the difference.

Consider you were just by ONE degree off when you are trying to cross the Pacific ocean in order to reach a specific island. Just that one degree off your course and you will miss your destination by many hundreds of miles, as the dissonance becomes not only cumulative, but even exponential!

Now the saddest thing about the whole process is that there was nothing at ALL wrong with your original idea, or with you, for that matter.

If I may continue the ocean crossing metaphor, you are a good captain and your sail boat is stoutly built; perfectly capable of withstanding the storms of the journey. It is even equipped with all the equipment you need and all that's wrong, all it takes to "miss the destination by hundreds of miles" and declare the expedition to have been an entire failure and total waste of time is ONE instrument, such as the compass, being just EVER so slightly off its true.

Or it might have been the rudder that was not perfectly calibrated and aligned, or perhaps the steering wheel that did not transmit exactly the right instructions – see, all it takes is a tiny flaw just somewhere and the most wondrous of projects will implode and basically fail over the so called "long haul".

This is a veritable tragedy, because once we are right there at the end of a long journey, having worked so hard and to the very best of our abilities, haven given our time, energy, hearts and souls to a project, when it then falters, flounders and basically sinks like a lead duck, we are upset by this (and rightly so), so terribly disappointed, and we'll look for a scapegoat.

Usually, we look in all the wrong places.

We blame ourselves for being fools in "believing that this could be done".

We berate ourselves for even having believed that there was an island out there in the first place in our darkest hours!

And all it takes is a few repetitions and we're not even talking about ocean crossings anymore. We might be lucky if we have enough "self esteem" left after that to go back and forth across the Channel once in a while on a butter-and-tobacco run; but many excellent people literally end up all washed up on the shore and think it was because there's something terribly wrong with them and God themselves didn't want them to succeed.

Calibrating The Energy Of A Project

Now, what I propose we do instead is to check out our proposed projects up front and before we ever leave the safety of the harbour for real.

Contrary to public opinion, project success is NOT like winning a lottery or a hit and miss affair over which we have little if no control.

Projects, like people and trees, tides and storms have patterns and they follow the laws of nature, of the universe just the same as everything else.

We don't need to see a sunrise to be able to guess there will be another one – it's pretty

much taken for granted that there will be another day after this one.

You don't have to be a magical soothsayer to be able to accurately predict that at some point in the future, it will rain again – of course it will! Rain is one of those natural patterns that turns up eventually, unless you live in a desert where it never or rarely rains, and then you'd have to be pretty stupid to be sitting there after a few years and NOT work out that simple fact of nature!

Such it is with projects too – businesses of all kinds, artistic endeavours, even relationships if you will.

These things are not random lightning strikes but they all have a pattern in them, an innate existence which involves birth, growth, maturity and death or whatever metaphor you want to use for the life cycles of everything and anything at all, even if people try and forget this.

When we set to work with the energy of a project, we are directly calibrating ourselves to its own innate patterns.

Consciously we absolutely cannot predict the future and therefore we guess and worry and turn ourselves into knots of freaked out activity as we are facing "the unknown future" – but there's a lot more to us than consciousness alone, and that's a very good thing when we consider the complexities of a project from an idea until it is entirely spent. That could be many thousands of years and possibly even more, so that is SOME complexity.

Let me give an example.

Let's say you wanted to write a book as your project.

Now as soon as we consider this, clearly you don't just want to "write the book".

There's more to it than that.

People write books so that other people would read them; so writing the book is only the very beginning of this possibly huge timeline as the book gets edited, proofread, published, printed, distributed, advertised, bought, sold, passed along ...

Along the line it may turn into a movie and become this whole new entity that came from the book but now has a life of its own (Lord Of The Rings is a good example of this, as is Moby Dick and the many, many versions of Oliver Twist and The Mutiny On The Bounty, to name just a few).

It may spawn computer games, action figures, conventions – but the deal with each and every project is always that it starts with an idea in ONE SINGLE PERSON'S MIND.

Genesis – THE IDEA

Someone, somewhere along the line had the idea that it was a good idea to build pyramids.

Someone, somewhere, had an idea about the energy system and we still have versions of their maps today.

An idea is an entity.

When an idea is made, at the energetic levels something has come into being which was not there before.

You can call this something a "thoughtfield" if you will but this thoughtfield, this little erea (existing energetic reality) contains the seeds that will become a massive, rock hard pyramid that stands for 10,000 years – and drives millions of archaeologists absolutely crazy as they are trying to figure out what exactly those things are meant to be!

So, as we want to be practical, let us now consider your project, YOUR idea.

In a moment, I am going to ask you to "tell me about your idea".

Now, I am only writing this document and so strictly speaking, I'm not there to listen when you do BUT – a great many people never get much beyond the ideas stage because THERE IS NO-ONE WHO WANTS TO KNOW, NO-ONE WHO WILL TRULY LISTEN.

I'm afraid I cannot give you a mountain of "hard" statistical research data but can only speak from my personal experiences here, yet I know that unless there is an outlet for explaining the idea in words to someone else an energetic movement that is absolutely necessary for the next step in the development of the project will simply never come into being.

Now above, I caps-locked on the phrases "who wants to know" and "who will truly listen".

In the usual construct set up, designed to stifle individuality and progress in every shape or form and cripple us all, quite frankly, when someone says, "I have a wonderful idea", they are not met with joy – not by their boss, not by their inferiors, not by their wife, not by their parents.

Constructville is entirely designed around retaining the status quo AT ALL COST – keeping things the way they have always been.

No matter how otherwise loving and supportive, folk will immediately and reflexively try and put a dampener on someone who is all excited about a new idea – who needs it, who wants it, if it was any good, don't you think it would have been invented already? It'll never work. Why don't you do something more useful, plough a field or have another baby, that'll take your mind of this nonsense ...

This happens usually long before our excited idea person ever got to explain it properly.

And here we come to the main point about the energy situation of expressing an idea fully – you choke that off half way through and already, the energy flow is not what it was supposed to be, the process of creation itself is already handicapped enormously and whatever that idea had the potential to become, is already crippled, right there and then.

Of course, this is reflexively done because anything that isn't the status quo threatens the status quo and would entail change; and of course, change is something to be feared. After all, we're all perfectly comfortable in our old rut and learning something new, oh dear! Oh dear oh dear! We've build ourselves a comfortable nest here which doesn't challenge us, doesn't have anything in it we can't control or at least kid ourselves we can control it and hey – don't rock the boat ...

I'm going on about this at some length not just because I am wanting to motivate you to actually really do the "expressing of the idea" in a moment, but also because you may well have "parts" in your construct which fulfil the dampening function for you – even in the absence of a tutting mother or a disapproving spouse, an undermining teacher or a sarcastic elder. You could think of the original perpetrators, even though they may be long gone, as having become internalised and now it is US – we ourselves! – who are mindlessly and endlessly repeating the old. (See the Evil CD protocol for that particular process and how to reverse it.)

The excuse (and what miserable excuse THAT is!) which is usually given for such appalling and creativity-and-freedom destroying behaviour is that it is supposed to "protect us" from our own stupidity and illusions, delusions of grandeur, from the pre-supposed and inevitable crushing disappointment when we fail yet again and come crawling back with our tails between our legs, like the classic prodigal son who "learned the hard way" that it's pointless trying to do something different, something challenging, something new.

We are adults and we don't need such protection.

Free from all this contortion and nonsense, we have more than enough intelligence and experience to know ourselves full well when something works and when it doesn't, when something is dangerous and when it isn't, and to make decisions based on that – which I prefer to making decisions based on old wife's tales and ill-conceived mutterings by those who would feel threatened if anyone did indeed succeed.

So.

Let's talk about YOUR idea.

This is just the basic idea. It's a thoughtfield with information in it and all the potential in the universe to become real and manifest most beautifully.

In the idea lies the seed for change – big change or little change, it matters not as the ripples spread far and wide across time and space and touch many others who will in the future buy your shaver, your new fangled Hoover, read your book, attend your training, visit your website, look at your paintings or whatever it is that you are about to manifest into the universe, uniquely you and yours, and this was never there before you made it become.

As you consider this, and read my words here, and you feel a fear or a drawing back at the potential responsibility and the repercussions of your project for yourself, your direct environment and over time, for other people and THEIR respective environments, then please treat yourself for that fear RIGHT NOW and until your energy system runs clear and clean, your thoughts are rational once more and cleanly logical, your body feels relaxed and you are ready and willing to give your idea its birth – the genesis, the magic words when from an idea it becomes translated into our world.

This happens when you explain your idea to me.

Now.

Please tell me about your idea.

I want to know all about it.

I am ready and I am listening.

What is your idea?

Step 1 – My Idea Is ...

Important Notes On The Threshold Challenge

Here are some more ideas from me to you as to how to approach this threshold challenge.

At this point, it is perfectly alright for the idea to be a little unclear and nebulous – of course! It is not yet a fully fledged project. It is only just about to be born!

When a baby is born, you won't even know what the colour of their eyes will be at first and that's a fact. There are MANY things we don't know about a baby when it appears. But as it grows, we learn these things about the new human as they unfold, and thus it is with projects and ideas.

In the act of telling someone who is sincerely interested you are already beginning to learn more about the project. There will be some things you are already perfectly clear about, others are still nebulous as I said, but it doesn't matter at this stage.

Tell ME everything about the project.

Now, you cannot do this energetic move "in the head alone".

For the idea to transition as an energetic entity, you need to speak or write the words or find some other medium which can be shared with others to "express the idea" and literally midwife its transition from idea to a project-to-be.

So, you must do something physically here.

One option is to imagine I am in the room with you and to tell me out aloud about your project. You can be absolutely assured that I will not laugh or think anything other than, "How amazing! Here is a person sharing an idea with me! How LUCKY am I to be here at this moment, at this so very special moment in time when this new project comes into this plane for the very first time!!!"

You can imagine my responses and my questions as I seek to find out more about it, and you can bet that I'll be excited about the project – if you are!

Allow yourself to be excited when you tell me or write to me what your idea is, in as much or as little detail as you can find within yourself.

If you have someone else you'd like to tell, then do tell them but please be careful.

Just "putting up with you" is NOT the conducive atmosphere for the birth of your project.

You absolutely need someone who is completely on your side for this one, so you can literally pour out your thoughts, your feelings, your ideas, free flowing mind storming expression – nothing held back, no holds barred, no shame or embarrassment at all, just pour it out.

You can do so in writing also but do it you must because it is then that we can truly begin to work with your energy and the energy of your project and adjust it here and now and before we do anything else at all.

One option that I have found really neat and helpful is to speak my words onto a tape recorder, pretending that there is an audience of one or many listening intently and really wanting to know all about the project who knew nothing about it yet. At first it was strange and hesitant, but then I really got into the flow of it and this is of course both perfect as a time saving device, as well as being perhaps the best option of them all to listen back to yourself and make notes.

You can further listen to disturbances in your voice, pick out incongruencies, places where you are being a little too vague or presuming too much.

ETPs can treat themselves for all manner of thoughts and feelings they are having whilst listening to the tape, including spotting Evil CDs, such as "Oh you have NO idea what you're talking about, do you." or "She'll never succeed," or "Ha! I've heard THAT before ... and remember times you've failed already? Well, ts, ts ...." – and so on and so forth.

Alternatively, note down any reservations, fears and objections whilst you are listening and treat these with EFT or any MET or approach of your choice.

The Project Energy

After you finished formulating your original outline, it is time to get magical.

Sit back, close your eyes if this helps and call up the project in your mind's eye.

What you will likely get at first is some "reality based picture" of the project – the book and its cover, the new shop, the town you are moving to, yourself counting the money happily you got from it or such.

- Although pictures say more than a thousand words, especially if they are movies, this is not information dense enough and relates to what we are doing here no more than looking at a little cartoon-coloured paper flyer for a circus relates to the experiences of going to a circus and living everything that happens on the night.

So we need to switch viewpoints now and consider the project as an energetic reality – and in doing so, dropping off the various pictures, sound tracks etc. and focussing on seeing and perceiving the energy of the project instead.

Use your hands to help you get a sense of where the project energy has formed as well as you reach out and touch the thoughtfield you have made and which contains all the available information and energy about our unfolding project for now.

A Note: If you haven't done this kind of energy work before, let me briefly remind us that when we switch to consider energetic realities, of course we still see some things but they do not represent as tables, books, chairs, lorries on streets or waving people.

They represent in much more basic and structural terms instead – such as a half formed globe, a dense field of different coloured sparkles, a smoky see through disc, a lattice of light or such.

This is essential in energy work because the "hard based" metaphorical representations, like a house, a book or a car, carry the wrong information or connotation which have come in from their "hard cousins" and the templates on which they are based and they distort our view of the energetic reality in many ways.

From the disturbances of old memories that are attached and the possibility of strong feelings which cause prejudices one way or the other and preclude clear thinking and interaction with the new thoughtfield, to the fact that a book is hard, requires gravity to work as a concept and also being rather static in time, these are all disturbances which get in between us and the energetic realities and confuse the issue terribly at this point.

Take your time over this experience and once again, I have found it extremely helpful to speak out aloud about the experiences or to write them down.

Remember that things done in the head alone are not as directly and powerfully linked to our actual reality experiences nor as clearly connected to our physical selves and the act of speaking or writing or both makes them much more real.

It gives you also much, much more leverage on interacting with your emerging entity as we can go back and re-read what we have written, or re-listen to what we have said if it has been recorded and thus gain a meta-position on what we are doing.

This further develops into a training record and contains many, many learnings for you personally, especially over time and when you know more about the processes and after you have done this many times all the way from the idea to full manifestation.

An Important Note: Remember that what we are doing here is not "just" about the one project we are doing right now; indeed, this is your first new project ever and although and as such you will always have a special place for this first process in your matrix ☺ and remember it with great fondness, we are indeed learning a process and a very powerful process at that which is entirely content free and will set you free to create whatever, whenever once you have learned it.

Make a note of your experiences as you touch the energetic reality that is your developing project in as much detail as possible.

Your First Unique Project Energy

Now, we have the project as an energetic reality right in front of you.

If it still seems a little nebulous, restart the original formation process with the words,

"Tell me more about it. I want to know MORE about it!"

... until the project is taking on an identity, and you can feel its own unique energy.

Let's pause for a moment so I can say to those who have actually done this now,

"Congratulations!"

Do you know how very few people even ever get this far?

Sure, it isn't their fault because we weren't taught how to do it and to make brand new projects is virtually forbidden – well, actually forbidden and heavily penalised, at that.

Of the few that get to express their idea and move it into this stage of existence, many people rush into a half formed project and try to make it work.

This, as you can imagine, is fraught with problems of all kinds and this is THE major single reason for projects getting bogged down and stuck beyond redemption somewhere further along the line.

For a project to flow and really work it needs to help you with its own energy and existence.

Any project derived from one of your own ideas becomes an energetic entity with a life and energy of its own that attracts things in its own right and does its own thing.

A project is not like a big lifeless rock that YOU have to lug forward at all but indeed an interactive event that generates power for its own purposes – from enthusiasm in you as you look at it grow and develop and which pulls you forward quite irresistibly right down to giving you interactive warning signs when things are going off balance and off kilter so you can calibrate to make it work correctly again.

This is exactly what artists talk about when they say that their project gives them life and provides them with energy – that is what projects are supposed to do!

They help you generate all the power you need to from your end, actively do what needs to be done to move it on and make it grow AND – they give you a surplus!

This surplus might come in the way of money, or attention, admiration, simply feeling happier in yourself or all of those – either way, your project is alive and you need to let it help you every step of the way as much as you help it to grow.

If at this point you need to refine your project a little more to make it come to life a little more so that it is quite real and you can feel its energy right there, please do so.

You might like to give your project A GIFT – indeed, one of the greatest and most powerful gifts to give it is to tell it out loud and clearly that "I have FAITH in you!"

This is an energy form which will literally light up your project, make it more powerful, and thus it becomes ever more real.

You & Your Project

Now, I want you to relax and simply call up your project so it is right in front of you and consider it, make contact with it.

Extend your conscious energy field so you can touch it and information is exchanged at that level between you and it, so that you both get to know and understand what each needs from the other to support them.

Particularly, I want you to pay very close attention to any problems from your end.

Are there shields, no matter how nebulous, remaining between you and your project or is "the air sparkling clear"?

Are you holding back somewhere?

Is there any part of you that is backing away, has reservations about the project, doesn't like it?

If so, of course this will create a dissonance between you and the project and as direct result, it can never become what it was truly meant to be – so sort it out!

Do you feel any blockages, old hurts or injuries in your body which would preclude a smooth and loving flow of energy from you to the project and back again?

Make especially sure that you do NOT fall back into the "one way street" service thinking which has been the bane of human children since the dawn of time – the mother "sacrificing herself" and being miserable, but rejecting all the energy and offers of return from the children at the same time.

Applied to a project and you'll get a stone you will have to lug uphill with ne'er a rest nor hope of it getting any better, so make sure you sort out the receiving end.

Where does this energy from the project come into me? What happens to it? Is it blocked? Is it running smoothly?

The energy from the project, remember, has at least a double function – it is of course to feed you in return (for projects are indeed generators!) but with the energy also comes information ABOUT the project.

The Magical Project Feedback Mechanisms

Let me repeat something very important from the last paragraph.

As you exchange energy with the project, you will of course also receive information about the project in return.

This information is absolutely essential for you.

Here is why:

It tells you things about the project you had not yet consciously noticed; but more, it is your feedback device, your control panel with flashing warning lights, status bars and all the levers necessary to correct things should they go astray.

It will let you know when the project needs what from you and in what measure; if you are doing something that is unhelpful or disturbing, the project will let you know through this exchange link right away and in return, as you are refining your hopes and plans for and with the project, it gets to know what you expect of it and can adjust likewise.

Problems With The Project

When I first started talking about this, one of the naysayers immediately said, "BUT (oh! THAT word! The naysayer's favourite spanner into your energetic works! Guaranteed to produce instant psychological reversal!) – "BUT - what if the project is a damp squib from the start? If it was never meant to be in the first place? If it really is a totally stupid idea?"

I replied, "Should that be the case it will probably manifest to you as a nasty glob of slime, a shardy spiky heap of mess or a painful ball of black-red fire puss. If, after three days of doing serious EmoTrance it still looks and feels like that and it hasn't gotten any better, then yeah, sure. Back to the drawing board of good ideas."

Frankly, I cannot even begin to conceive of anyone having what they consider to be a "good idea" and it manifesting like this!

What is much more likely is that your project as a whole feels and appears really nice but it might have a dark spot somewhere, something sticking out that doesn't belong, or there's simply a sense of dissonance or there being something not quite right with it.

Now this is not a sign of failure but instead, we'll jump up and clap our hands in delight and say, "Wow! Thank GOODNESS!!! I noticed that right now and here and I can do something about it this very instant! How WONDERFUL to be able to adjust the project at this level, so easily and perfectly, and without wasting years chasing my tail when unexpected problems keep creeping in later in the reality stage for seemingly no good rhyme or reason!"

What we will do is to extend to the project, link up with it in conscious awareness and literally and simply, soften and flow the trouble spots so they may find their rightful place – either as a part of the project, or their rightful place may be somewhere else that has nothing to do with it.

Here are some other ideas for project trouble-shooting at this stage.

I've already mentioned The Gift. Asking the project what it needs from you is one way of finding just the right energy to balance and stabilise it, to bring it into harmony with yourself.

Another version is to simply let your so called "intuition" decide on a gift for the project. You may absolutely use the metaphor container to deliver the medicine if you will :-) – your project might need a flower, or perhaps some precious metal, sunshine, birdsong – whatever it is, provide it and take it from there.

Distance and detachment. A great many of us are reluctant to get "wholeheartedly" involved with a new project because of past trauma, failure and pain and so we might keep the project at arm's length, if you will – when the perfect distance in real terms might be half an arm's length or less. Also, and this is the next point, I would mention again ...

Shields. To make this work you have got to drop shields to the project entirely and let it connect with your heart. Alright, so I'll use the phrase – you've got to allow yourself to love your project because it needs that to grow strong and bring you benefits and support you wanted it for all along. You need to really treat yourself for any fears or reservations which may remain.

Please do not worry that you are tapping or ETing "well founded fears" away when you do this. As you grow calm and stable in yourself, you might even find your inner eyes and sense opening to some aspect of the project you had not hitherto noticed and which indeed, requires attention.

Those are never found nor seen if fear remains and so they cannot be corrected and become the reason for the project to be much more difficult in the end that it ever need have been.

Fine Tuning Your Project

Now, and still and "only" working with energetic entity that is your project, we are going to take some time to really get to know it, to live with it for a while and to fine tune ourselves and it as information flows between the two of us.

I suggest you allow a week for this, calling your attention to the energetic entity of your project every so often and in different states and circumstances.

The thing is that your project has to be in tune with all of you – not just "you on your good days" when you are feeling positive, proactive and enlightened.

This project is, let us remember, a source of energy and a most helpful addition to your life and energy system and it's an unconditional deal – warts and all if you will.

This also gives you the opportunity to discover more blockages, injuries and problems along the line which would otherwise not have become apparent. See, when you are all happily balanced and relaxed, that's nice and energy flows freely, but when you're upset or angry or afraid, THAT is when you have access to these old injuries that are still causing troubles and WILL continue to cause problems in the future – unless YOU do something about them and sort yourself out.

Really do your best to remember, even in the pits of depression, that your new project is here to HELP YOU most specifically and in a way that no human or pet ever could and to allow it to support you as you discover your blockages, reversals, shields and injuries and go about resolving and repairing those.

As you are doing this, you will also consciously become aware of how much more you already KNOW about your project now – even though beyond speaking or writing the original idea we have done no goal setting, planning or anything else for that matter.

You might also find during this time that there are already unexpected happenings coming your way as a result of your energy work on the project and on yourself.

Be delighted when this happens and send a little loving to the energy system you are building here – and watch and feel it tingle back a charge of delightful energy in response!

When you are happy that your little baby energetic reality project is in tune with you (it doesn't have to be 100% perfect yet – indeed, it cannot yet be all it will become, it's a baby, remember? :-) and your relationship is mostly dissonance free, we can take the next step in bringing it into this plane.

Step 2 – Me & My Project

Write down or speak aloud on tape, then make notes on your relationship with your project, what you did exactly to make these even better all around, and what you learned as a result.

Also include what your project now appears like when you describe it as an energetic reality.

The Project Identity

Now's the time to name your project.

It will be given a real name, like a word – the name of your new company, the title of your new book or album or painting, the title of your training and so forth.

But what we will also do, is give it a symbol.

Symbols are pretty powerful things when they are done right and used correctly and we shall do both. It isn't actually at all as difficult as the muttering old folks will have you believe (mostly to keep you from doing it, and thus being able to affect real CHANGE!) and well worth doing.

Chances are that most of you reading this will readily have a name and a symbol come to them.

It is really simple thus naming an energetic reality of your own making (!!) that you have a flow of contact, energy exchange and information with – the project will literally tell you its own name.

If you are not sure, try some things.

It will guide you even in the most basic of yes-no, hot-cold responses in the right direction.

On the symbol front for example, you could pay attention to your project and suggest that the symbol should be a square.

You'll get an instant kinaesthetic answer to that one and you can work your way towards the conscious breakthrough moment of knowing exactly what the symbol should be quite quickly.

- *WARNING!* Do not let anyone else make this symbol or the name for your project. This is YOUR project and it belongs to you in all ways, it is a part of YOUR energy system.

I really don't care if the greatest prophet of all ages materialises on your doorstep and tells you convincingly he's found the right name for your project straight out of the Akashic records – your own words and symbols have the power, YOUR power and they will be righter than anything anyone else can give you.

Please also do NOT use a stock symbol such as a pentagram or a ying-yang circle or such.

Pre-used public stock symbols can NEVER, NEVER be the right symbol for your unique and brand new project and carry with them basically the shit and misconceptions, the misuse and lies perpetrated over the ages under its innocent name. If you are desperate for something very like a stock symbol, say a pyramid, then make sure to put a nose, a couple of ears and a tail on it so it is your own and immediately recognisable by all concerned as basically, NOT A PYRAMID any longer at all!

* *An Important Note:* I cannot overstate the importance of this to keep your Project Energy safe and right; but although this is incredibly serious, it is also a great deal of fun and not at all difficult.

See, a squiggly line with a curly tail or simply a few dots is all that is required and this has just absolutely nothing to do with your perceived artistic or creative talents. If you need help with this step which in spite of the powerfields of the ages is the simplest of all human endeavours, please use any energy therapy form to clear fears or misconceptions, and remember the thought flow process as well as an alternative to have ideas delivered straight from your energy mind if necessary – it knows best!

The Project Messengers

The symbol and the name, wherever they are placed, become links to your project – like spider strands. As the symbol and name are of the project and entirely unique, wherever they ever are, they serve to evoke the project and its energy absolutely specifically. Think of it as the energetic equivalent of the unique file locator system on the Internet. There may be many billions of files but it is organised so that no two files can possibly have the same address and thus cause misunderstandings and confusion.

The symbol and the name become interchangeable and recognisable for the project itself.

Thus, someone browsing a magazine that may have an advertisement with your project's title and logo will be able to tune into the project from their end and understand what it is about in essence immediately.

It will jump off the page at them and actively draw their attention because it is real, it is live and has been made in cohesive volition.

This is incredibly magical as you can imagine and very, very powerful indeed, even on your very first time out as a true energy magician.

It is simply so that most people who make names and logos TRY for this kind of thing but ...

- a) Don't really know what exactly they're supposed to be doing or what it's for;
- b) Often rely on stock symbols whose power is so diffused now by misuse, they might as well not bother (such as the yin/yang

for example that is literally splotched on every other mind/body/spirit type advertisement!); and

c) Because their projects have never been properly refined nor energised as we have done/are in the process of doing.

Attracting The Right Energies In Return

Whilst we're on the topic of "symbols jumping off the page with power" and "people being able to tune into the entity that is the project" – of course, this is also very practically what brings the exactly right people to you as a result.

This is the mysterious "drawing the right people towards you" as opposed to blindly chasing around in a crowded market place, trying to catch the slower ones who couldn't get away in time in your net and dragging them towards your product whilst they kick and scream!

Your project, having a clear and well defined energetic reality of its own now, is a veritable beacon, a lighthouse if you will, amidst the general confusion and lack of clarity in the construct world.

Now finally, here's something that feels right, it's powerful.

There are no lies here, no false promises.

This product is what it is, it's not trying to fool anyone or pretend to be more or better or more valuable – it is a clear, clean, shining thing in harmony with its creator.

Step 3 – Your Project's Identity

Describe the process by which you derived the special name.

Describe the process by which you derived the symbol for your project.

Write down your project's special name and draw its special symbol and any notes on the topic you might like to add.

The Naming Ceremony

Ah yes, it is time to really get magical again and bring it all together in a much improved, fully refurbished and advanced progression of the ancient and highly revered event that is "The Naming Ceremony".

Hereby we call up our project and officially give it its name and its symbol.

By now, I think we have all understood that this is not just happening in the mind space but we have to do so properly and with physical actions involved; now it is getting really real!

Now, we have a small drawing of your symbol with the name written underneath for real and present in the Hard.

And this is what we do.

We hold the paper with the drawing and the name in both hands, hold it to our hearts.

Tune in to your project and make full contact, until you are full of love and absolutely delighted by the interaction between you, the flow of energy and charge as you exchange information and states of being, pure energy too. By all means, allow yourself to enjoy this, to be excited by it in a very physical sense, very emotional if you want or need – that's all perfectly alright.

Then simply let words come to you when you're ready, perhaps something to this effect:

"Darling, dearest project, beloved child of my mind, my body, my heart and soul, I officially welcome you with the greatest joy – awaken in my life and come into being!

Your name is (...) and this is your very own special symbol by which all will recognise you!"

"Welcome To The World!"

Now, I've done this myself and I really can tell you, it's a most extraordinary experience which you must really allow to flow right through you in all ways – it feels like something is really being switched on, it feels great!

Allow yourself to experience this fully and know that your Project Energy (which you from now on call by its special and unique name – but as I don't know this here, can you make the mental adjustment and use your own project's name for now in that place!) has given you its very first gift.

Here, for the first time you have absolute proof in the most incontrovertible way that your project has something incredibly important to give TO YOU and will continue to do so for as long as your relationship and its own life cycle continues.

Please make sure you receive this gift (that charge experience as the threshold shift occurs in response to you having named and officially welcomed your project) in the right spirit and correctly, namely by allowing it to enter your heart and letting it flow all the way through you and out, changing you in the process.

It is such a wonderful clear and innocent energy form and so very personal at that, of course there is the temptation-reflex of the old to hold on to it and make it into a Guiding Star but that is NOT the point and should you do that, it will tie you unhealthily to that one project forever and a day.

No! It must FLOW because it is the FIRST and NOT the only one and that is how it should be, must be for all to proceed correctly and unfold just as it should for both of you. There's nothing as miserable a sight as a creator dragging around their dusty, long gone past project because they made a Guiding Star when it was born by accident and now cannot let go of it, nor understand just why it is that they cannot re-live its glory – and worst of all, can't understand why nothing like that has ever "happened to them" again or since that day!

These things cause "creator's blockage" in humans and that's not what we want or need; if necessary, bundle the whole experience up in a Snow Globe and very deliberately pass it on to the higher processing systems for proper storage.

I really can't emphasise strongly enough how important this is to have YOU understand this for me; because the Guiding Star formation to the energy of a project, especially in this early stage, will also inexorably lead to the project not being able to grow and develop any further as well

– and thus it never reaches its maturity, its wonderful potential, gets tied back in time to this baby state and all it could have been is lost.

But back now to our Naming Ceremony. We have connected to our project, spoken the words of welcome and dedicated the name and symbol and in return, experienced the threshold shift as it was "born into this plane" – this was the project's gift for us.

Now it is time to give the project a gift in return. In human baby ceremonies, the idea is to give the new arrival something they'll need to thrive in this new plane and therefore, changed environment.

It is completely logical that our little energy baby product too will now require something else from you that it didn't require when it was still altogether of the energetic planes and before we called it to be here in physicality as well.

As a swift aside :-) this adjustment step is the falling hurdle for the good people you might have met who always have amazing ideas – but they don't work in practice, quite mysteriously! It all becomes so straightforward if you take the planes of energy and mind and put them back together with physicality events in the right order and sequence, it is sometimes quite ridiculous when one considers how many good people "fail" or drive themselves crazy, time and time again, simply because they were never told and did not know about this.

And so, to your gift for your project.

This is a gift of energy of course because at this stage, our project is still nearly entirely of energy and nothing much aside, apart from your notes and its name and symbol on paper. It still eats energy and needs energy to thrive right now.

However, the Gift is and has always been closer to physicality than just being entirely of the energetic realms because it uses metaphoric representations of physical objects, such as trees, landscapes, specific colours, objects and such.

Now, and ONLY AFTER you have created and run your ceremony, we give a physical type gift to our little project. As always with such things, consciously we really couldn't begin to work out what it needs so once again you'll have to let something come to you.

Be relaxed about it and easy and something will appear. And don't be afraid of doing this wrong. You have a really powerful connection to your project and it'll really let you know if you pick the wrong thing right away and try to feed it something poisonous, destructive or unhelpful by accident.

Also, and as this isn't a standard limited old ceremony at all, by all means give more than one gift if that feels good and your project is asking for it.

One or many, remember to speak it out aloud as you transfer the gift as well. If it comes too swiftly and is too swiftly ingested by your project, don't worry and just change the tense; instead of "I give you the gift of (....) with all my heart" as you would say during the transfer, you can simply say, "I gave you the gift of (....)!" and have a laugh instead.

I would strongly advise you to then take a moment just to be with your project, enjoy it, love it, interact and play with it – I use the term to "dance with it" because I often literally get up and have a dance with the erea in question, simply because it feels right and is so enjoyable.

This concludes the strictly necessary parts of the naming ceremony; these are the main components once more in brief:

The Naming Ceremony Step By Step
1. Connect with your project energy.
2. Hold the name and symbol to your heart.
3. Speak the name and declare the symbol out aloud.
4. Officially welcome the project to the world.
5. Receive your gift from the project and let it flow through you.
6. Give your welcome gift to the project in return and declare this out aloud.
7. Take a moment to "dance with your newly born project energy" in delight.

You can do the ins and outs and create the scenes and surrounds for these basic steps any way you like. From simply sitting at your desk and doing it there in the course of your everyday work, to inviting a horde of friends for a feast and naming party and dancing into the night via putting on some happy music, lighting some candles and putting out some flowers in acknowledgement of the event, how you frame this it is entirely up to you in all ways.

One thing though – have it be right for you and have it be FUN. Indeed, this is central to the whole deal and so here is ....

***** *An Especially Important Note:* For the love of the Creator, please DON'T approach this step with the dour misery and black magic mindset of spookiness nor even the severe harshness or serious holiness of "religious ceremonies" you might have encountered in the past.

Those were the old, this is the new and here we do such things VERY differently.

We do these things in a spirit of love and fun, with lightness and delight, in excitement and joy, knowing in every fibre of our beings that this our birthright, making use of a simple ability the creator itself gave US for a wonderful gift and we are exercising this for the first time, flexing our little wings and beginning to learn to fly.

Come on guys, this is fun! You have a baby energetic entity which you are blessing whilst holding a piece of paper to your heart! This is lightness, this is delight, this is a WONDERFUL welcome ceremony, just exactly what a baby's naming and arrival-welcome party should be like!

This is exciting, this is HAPPINESS.

And which is why there is no need to cast circles "for protection from the dark forces which may lurk and pounce" or any of that at all. Why you can do it anywhere, any time, with full waking awareness and right there in body and in mind.

And why you may really want to celebrate this in any way you want – with music, with a feast, with a dance or by opening a bank account for your baby – please yourselves once the ceremony has been accomplished!

Assistance, Guidance and Conditions

Now we have a centrally important stage of this wonderful Project Energy game.

Please note that we have not set any goals, have not put any pressure on the project of any kind – this entire deal has been about you and the project and nothing else besides.

Of course, the time comes for your project to reach out and interact with others in many different ways. May these others be suppliers, supporters, customers or helpers of whatever kind, they too will have to engage with the project on many levels and in many different ways to get that reality ball rolling, as they say in the trade.

A lovely young man with a mother who holds a machete and snarls insanely puts off the most eager of suitresses indeed, so here too it is not just about the project itself but also about what YOU bring to the unfolding party event so that the energy exchanges must flow smoothly and delightfully.

Your project is innocent and sparkling bright, now let's make sure that we don't get inadvertently in its way in any way whatsoever, and that we can deal with the interactions which must arise most smoothly.

Let's start with the intended recipients.

Recipients & Facilitators

Sometimes, a project is about selling something directly to customers or wholesalers, other times there are other kinds of facilitators needed along the line, such as agents and publishers for example which must connect and resonate in perfection with your project for it to become as it should.

Once again, let us call up your project (you now do so by name directly or by symbol!).

When you are fully aware of your standing joyful resonance connection and you are more or less of one and the same mind, we call up the recipients and facilitators.

So, whoever you intend to present your project to for the usage or decision on furthering of, call them up and tune into their respective fields.

A Note: It is absolutely fascinating how this simple manoeuvre actually outperforms classic paper and pencil market research every time (if done correctly!) and how it provides information that ordinary marketing research techniques simply do not have access to. And more fun still, this exercise can actually tell you directly if you have major misconceptions which would indeed need further research to rectify before we go any further!

Here are some questions that will have to be addressed.

- Is your "market" or intended recipients and facilitators clear? Is it nebulous? If so, what do you have to do to make it become more cohesive?

- How does your own energy system respond as you are reaching out and connecting with these groups of people or individuals?

- What needs to be done to get all of this – the you/project unit and the market – to resonate harmoniously?

There are some core occurrences in this exercise which can be quite challenging.

For one thing, there may be a LOT of prejudice in you about your market (and please remember I am using this term for anyone and everyone who comes into contact with your project, audience, customers, facilitators, bystanders, reviewers, critics, reporters etc. etc. etc.).

You might think certain people are not interested because in the past you've never found a way to explain yourself to them in such a way that they would understand.

You might have deliberately excluded some segments of your natural market for personal past injury reasons. This is, by the way, far more common than you might believe – for example, I once knew a holistic healer woman who, after having been very badly treated by her then boyfriend, turned all her practice related doings bright pink and covered with fairies, teensy angels and dolphins; began to more or less exclusively invoking "the goddess energy" – and thus structurally and

VERY practically reducing the amounts of men in her workshops and healing practice to ZERO.

There may be segments of your market you simply don't understand at all because you never had contact with them but heard bad things being said about "their kind"!

Whatever you find, and whatever reasons you have had in the past to produce blockages, shields, reversals, barriers and veritable minefields between yourself and your markets, sort them out.

The same goes for any past occurrences which are still causing ripples in the flow, such as past failures and disappointments with a seemingly similar project (note! SEEMINGLY!).

Remember – THAT was the old.

This IS the new and here, we are different, we do things differently.

Be bold.

Do this part of the exercise boldly and in as much depth, for as much length as you need to until you really have a flow established between you/your product and the market, the true give-and-receive flow in one single movement which is what carries the information we require.

Should you fall away or into doubt at any point during this part of the unfoldment, centre on your heart and start from there, again.

Project Adjustments

This contact with the market field might well necessitate some change to you and to your project. Indeed, if it did not I would be most surprised indeed!

Your project's environment now, that it is here amongst us, absolutely includes the market and if you have ever partaken of the nature VS nurture debate, then you will be aware just how profoundly the environment shapes the original intention.

Now, the challenge lies in both allowing the interaction with the market to perform the very necessary function of letting your project know how it is to thrive under these environmental conditions and at the same time and in exactly the same place, for YOU to retain exactly the loving connection to your project you experienced when first it was conceived, then born.

This is a truly magical balance which marketers the world over and through all times of human trades and projects have sought as their holy grail – namely how exactly to have a product that doesn't become distorted as the creator "tries to feed the taste of the market" and in doing so, destroys all that was ever valuable and good about it; nor on the other hand, end up with a project that may be cohesive still but is completely, totally and utterly rejected by the market!

In the worlds of hard, this is indeed a challenge and possibly even an impossible paradox – art vs. the market, if you will.

In the elegant worlds of energy however, it is easy to do as there is so much more flexibility; but further, here we are setting the intention of the project and believe it or not, the intention of the project is what draws or repels the market rather than its content, structure or physical manifestation in the end.

It is my contention that a project without a market is a fish without water – they are part of one and the same meta-system and must by needs, flow and function together and in harmony, the market explaining its needs and the project filling these with itself; in return, the project explaining its needs and the market giving the project what it needs to grow.

Remember, my phrasing of market is not just about buying customers.

Projects might need all sorts to grow.

They might need a champion who speaks up for them, they might need people talking about it to start to glow; they might need synchronicities, good fortune, luck or whatever you might want to call it; gifts from the market and then of course, "hard food" in the form of money to help it grow.

So what we have here is once again, an Even Flow of change and of momentum.

This interaction with the market will and should change your project considerably in many different ways; and for us as the creators it is essential we should not now go all Guiding Star on the original idea or baby project and try and hold that unfoldment back in any shape or form.

"Oooh but it was so pure and sweet when it was new" is an unhealthy attitude to any child and it is of course for our project – remember I said right at the beginning that we can't even know yet what it might become?

Get your energetic balancing with the market right and it will ALWAYS remain pure and sweet – even when it is being investigated by the trusts and mergers commission in 12 years from now!

Many artists and healers and such think that the market tries to break their projects, prostitute them, make them into pap for the lowest common construct denominator but that is actually entirely untrue.

It works out like that in the end because there was no clear energetic cohesion between creator-project-market from the start but instead a lot of negativity, dissonance and disturbances all around which were never addressed and got worse and worse as the project tried to grow – and that's when "Mickey Mouse grows up a cow" and Mozart starves to death in his attic. Of course, once HE was out of the equation, people were then set free to celebrate the very beautiful projects he had assembled ... ah the mystery of the starving artists of the ages, finally resolved ... :-)

At the energetic level, you can recognise that the mysterious market is not a pile of evil stupid constructs, but indeed, energetic entities with very real needs which, if your project interacts correctly and "in the right spirit" to fill them with its unique essence, will lead to very real exchange-rewards for the project in return quite naturally and simply because that is how it was supposed to be.

A Little Note: I, Silvia, very personally, have my disturbances in the flow exactly at this point. You can tell this exactly by the way this chapter-step is just not flowing as the others did, it has more words, it isn't as light or joyful as the ideas chapter, or loving or naming your project.

But don't let MY personal quirks on the topic of the creator-project-market energy balancing allow you to in any way forget the sense of lightness and of fun that needs to be here.

Even though I'm still having problems with this (which will soon be resolved, I promise to all who may be listening!) as I write this, I know exactly what I need to look for.

Instead of wrestling through sleepless nights with markets, repercussion, accusations, and all sorts of old stuff, I need to learn to dance joyously and delightedly with the market – for all concerned in this party with the project the star guest but without creator and market present, not much of an event at all!

So, let's get to work in this spirit of "being determined to have fun" LOL and get balancing, why don't we!

Step 4 – Creator-Project-Market Balancing

Call up your project, then your project's respective market. How do they appear to you?

Now, take 3rd party position on the C-P-M triad which includes you as well and from here, do what needs to be done to establish a perfectly even flow between all three systems. What are you discovering as you do this?

You can switch viewpoints into each one of these to do repair work or adjust things or to understand each better. What insights did this give you?

Note how all three change as they begin to interact systemically and as they should. How has the system changed? How does it now appear to you?

Getting Practical

That's a bit of joke because how much more practical can you get than to align a project in this way before we start hiring casts of hundreds and spending thousands on advertising?

But what I mean by that is that practically, you have a new challenge.

This project is already more alive and familiar to you than probably anything else you've done before and for good reason – what we were always doing blindly, half unconsciously and hindered by a total lack of understanding of the energetic processes involved in genesis, has been approached in a simple and intuitive way and your project is named, close to your heart and resonating harmoniously, providing you with energy and information about itself as it grows.

Bringing in that dimension of not just you and your project, but in the context of the C-P-M triad single system, you will absolutely already know far more about marketing your project and to whom than probably anyone ever did on this planet.

I bet you can't wait to get started!

The new challenge is to learn to do your "practical" business planning in a whole new way and to stop yourself from falling back into the old ways which led you – here.

By this I mean if you find yourself all of a sudden doing some quota forecasts, goal setting or filling in a business plan or doing all and any of the things you used to think were necessary or essential – STOP.

The energy system that is the triad is now going to kick in as most helpful in providing feedback as to what is useful within its own context, and what isn't.

If a business plan just happily flows from the tip of your pen and upon tuning into your projects' field you find it is most delighted and growing as you write, then yes, we do a business plan.

If upon checking back with the true essence of the triad you find it has gone dark, drawn further away, is swirling helplessly or just basically screams, NOOO!!! then stop it.

That's of the old, and we're in the new.

Here, things are done VERY differently.

Here, we take advice from the triad system itself.

What is the next step?

Now I know that actually physically asking the project or the market or even yourself is basically never necessary because if information is flowing all the time between you and it and them, of course you will know what the triad needs – you can feel it, see it, see it with your night eyes, sense it, feel it right in your own body.

Not only will you know WHAT to do but also when, in which order and sequence and even HOW as you simply flow with the unfoldments of the triad.

You might find out that for the triad system to function most efficiently, it needs something from you that you do not yet have – the freedom to speak truthfully in public, for example or the ability to pick up a telephone and make a pitch to a stranger; it is up to you to fulfil your part of the relationship to enable the triad itself to help you further.

This is, of course, information exchange and processing of an order as we might have rarely, if ever, experienced before and more different from reading advice in a book on business than space travel is from self mutilation.

Our job as conscious selves is to get hold of this information now and take the necessary physical steps for which you need a physical body – such as picking up the phone to order some brochures, or typing out an advertisement or such.

And in order to consciously know what we're supposed to be doing next, we are going to what I can only think of calling "channelling".

Only, we're not channelling from some strange alien entity with a weird name which may or may not exist at all, but indeed, we are going to channel from our own energy mind, previously known as the "unconscious mind" because they couldn't see it, which has all the available data on everything now – on the market, on the project and on YOU (!!) and how it all interacts.

If you have never done this like this before – and who has? I certainly haven't! – it may feel just a little bit peculiar to be passing over such "hard" things as whether to buy pencils first with your project's name on it or whether to talk to the architect instead to the energy mind.

But frankly, who else could possibly compute this level of complexity?

We've always known that "we" as in who we thought we were without such superb devices as the energy mind at our disposal couldn't possibly handle all of that – and we were absolutely right.

Now, "channelling" information, and never mind completely rock hard information about stationary and book-keeping is all about opening the communication channels between our conscious minds and our energy mind which has this information all ready and worked out, in the precise order and sequence.

It may take a little practice as how to not:

a) Expect channelling to be mysterious, Oracle-of-Delphi-like nonsense;

b) Get in the way with conscious thought whilst channelling is in process and thus disturb and confuse the flow of information (which tends to lead to oracle-of-Delphi type nonsense!);

c) Be all tense and distrustful at the process, thinking the energy mind "only knows metaphors" or such.

Traditionally, we make a record of channelling anything because it can flow very fast plus at the beginning it is hard to remember everything because it involves a state shift.

If you can "channel and type" like me, doing this on a keypad in real time is a good option. If you can take down notes and channel at the same time, you can do that. If you find it difficult to "channel and type" at the same time, then you MUST use a tape recorder for now because you need a record of what was said and revealed to check over after the fact.

*** A Note:*** When you later go over your own "channelled" materials, make a note to look for the places where you can really see/notice/feel that there was the energy mind at work, and where you were being consciously trying to be helpful.

This is really very useful at the beginning and as we are practically learning something which is both very human as well as so rare that the folk who can do it well get given Pulitzer and Nobel prizes ...

By all means, before you have your very first ever Project Energy channelling session which will reveal to you the steps you have to take, in real linear time, in absolute practical physicality, to continue the growth and flow of the total triad, treat yourself for any reservations, fears, misconceptions.

By all means make sure you're as clear and joyful as can be, light and enthusiastic, intrigued by the whole proposition and absolutely willing to stumble a bit as any beginner would when they first learn the moves of a new game.

By all means, hold firmly in the back of your mind the thought that whatever happens, it'll get better and better with just a little practice – and with a deep breath and a smile, let us now:

Step 5 – The First Practicals

Contact the C-P-M triad directly. Hold it clearly in your attention, and from this overview position, dive right into the system until you are one and the same with it.

Sit yourself down in front of a typewriter, keyboard, note pad or tape recorder, and basically, now "channel" the requisite first steps for you to take in physicality.

Remember to look at this as a game and allow yourself to be completely surprised by what you end up writing or saying.

So let's find out! What do you need to do next?

The Journey Has Begun ...

So then, here we are.

Young ones if you will, bright and new, beginning to play the old games in a whole new way.

What's next?

I'm sure I don't have to tell you this, really, It is obvious and flows logically from all we have talked about and done before we got to this point.

Now, we allow the journey of the triad to unfold.

This is a dance and path which has a power all of its own and this is what makes it so new and so absolutely exciting of course – WE do no longer have to do all the work ourselves, think and plot and plan ourselves into exhaustion but instead, here is an event taking place because of us, coming from us and through us alright but we're not alone.

We are a part of a supporting triad which benefits all around and gets stronger, more loving and simply more fantastic and ALIVE as it goes along.

Ok, so we are young and new to all of this, and I wouldn't have lived the old for as long as I have if I wasn't thinking now that "it can't possibly be as simple as this!" or "You better write something motivational for when things go horribly wrong so they don't lose heart ..."

Oh sod that, as they say in the UK!

NOTHING can go wrong in a true unfoldment, because if it is unfolding, then it is perfect, and that's really as simple as that.

In the old, when we hit a brick wall, we bashed our heads against it until it hurt and bled; in the new, we flow around it as though it wasn't even there, changing direction with ease, not having to prove anything to anybody any longer and without a second thought because the flow itself is the delight, IS the joy.

I don't think any of us even need to be told that having a standing resonance connection with the triad system is the key and core; that is the feedback device and the navigation instrument constantly at work, always there, guiding the unfoldment from within itself, always in joy and in confidence.

As long as we are willing to play our part from our end, and until we decide to do something else instead or create other, new projects, this triad system will flow and produce the goods for all and everyone who is involved in it.

Is THIS what "they" actually try for when they talk about "win-win-win" situations?

☺

Project Energy Conclusion – And Some Metaphysical Musings ...

So, what we have here is for us to simply take our ability to create an energy system literally out of nowhere :-) just by willing it to be so.

We have found out that this energy system – the C-P-M triad – is actually and structurally designed to give YOU something you want and need and that basically cannot be had in any other way.

Relationships with self, soul, God, the Universe, family, kids and other people are one thing. A relationship with something you have created yourself and sharing it with others is another altogether. It is something that true adults do.

It is most likely, structurally built into us to WANT to do this – much like ferrets can't stop trying to dig even when they're caged on steel, really.

People can't stop trying to create things.

Oh but how the "powers that be" have tried to stop them in every way possible – entrainment, undermining, punishment, putting the fear of God in them, withdrawing love and attention, incarcerating and even burning them – and still, people just don't seem to be able to stop!

I think we do it because we can, and also and much more importantly, because in the process of doing it, we are learning something, bringing hitherto undiscovered and unexplored parts of our energy systems online and doing something very important indeed for the development into being a fully actualised human being.

This very simple set of making a project from an idea is indeed, what used to be called "High Magic" and guarded so ferociously over the ages, demonified and condemned – much like people's genitals, really, and both those and our ability to do magic were entirely built in and come as standard with the base model human being, courtesy of the Highest Creator themselves.

It is really inconceivable to me how something as natural and simple as this "Project Energy" set could have been so perverted, twisted, warped into some travesty of truth and basically destroyed across the ages by people who should have known better – but blatantly didn't.

It is entirely respectful of ourselves and of creation.

It is empowering, educational and entirely natural.

And chances are, it is a step stone without which we will NEVER find out what's beyond or WHY we made these projects and symbols, what exactly that energy is that we are getting from them, and more importantly still, what we are going to use the surplus energy provided by the C-P-M triad for in the long run.

Frankly, I dream of a world where people present their projects, and their projects are cohesive, honest, unique – oh, so desirable! What contributions these are!

I can't wait for yours. I raise a glass filled with sparkling, living energy to you in toasting your new projects – and mine.

Blessed you are,

Silvia Hartmann, July 2003

EmoTrance To Energy Magic: The Freedom Spells

My rage and my sorrow,

I now let you go –

Soften and flow,

Soften and FLOW!

This is a generally useful "release spell format" that works neurologically as well as on the energy levels.

It corrects faulty thinking and really gets the old energy system moving where it was previously stuck.

Freedom Spells actually correct structural problems between the conscious mind and neurological processing and the energy system long term, and by **LEARNING TO CORRECT MISTAKES AS THEY OCCUR IN REAL TIME.**

* Please Note: EmoTrance Is Required. First, you need to know and be able to do EmoTrance to work this, else it will remain nothing but meaningless words for the majority of people.

The Spell Format

Secondly, these things are WORDED IN SPELL FORMAT, i.e. a direct conscious instruction to the totality.

Hence it is simple, direct, it rhymes and it is really an instruction. Not a command, for the totality really doesn't deserve such treatments, but a CONFIDENT DIRECTION given by the conscious mind, as it can do by design.

The spell format is made up of PULSES OF ENERGETIC INFORMATION BEING TRANSMITTED, hence the rhythm and rhyme, and you will be able to feel how that is very, very different from a prayer or an affirmation in every way, and in personal experience.

Please bear in mind that the spell format can be used repeatedly – three's a charm, and if you want to say it in much the same way someone will flick their light switch 33 times so their family doesn't die, by all means, do it in a moment of crisis, because that WORKS TO KEEP US FROM GOING TOTALLY MAD when stress is high.

That's why these people do it!

Freedom Spells The Basic Instructions

To start this off, do it deliberately and in the Heart Healing posture, speaking the words out aloud and taking time to make sure that the very first three or four things really do "soften and flow" in response.

Your first attempts might need a bit of encouragement but that's just a part of the natural learning curve. Bear with it, it gets better fast.

After that, speak it out aloud and let whatever sequence of things wanting to be released slip slide off into the good old universal oceans of energy.

It is a highly addictive process that one instinctively seems to want to do more of and my advice is, just go for it and do it compulsively for a time until the PATTERN HAS BECOME ESTABLISHED and even in mid-speak, if you hear yourself say or think things like, "Oh this fucking idiot ..." and the echo comes INSTANTLY – "My rage and frustration, I now let you go - soften and flow, soften and flow!"

Freedom Spells - Examples

The spell has to work as a pulsing rhythm, so use words around the core instruction to make sure it does not stumble.

Here are a few examples of how to make the basic format work for different circumstances:

All of my sorrow
I now let you go
Soften and flow,
Soften and flow!

All the old definitions
I now let you go -
Soften and flow,
Soften and flow!

My mother's madness,
I now let you go,
Soften and flow,
Soften and flow!

All that still hurts me
I now let it go,
Soften and flow,
Soften and flow!

All my old grief,
I now let you go,
Soften and flow,
Soften and flow!

All of the past,
I now let you go,
Soften and flow,
Soften and flow!

All the ancient betrayals,
I now let you go.
Soften and flow,
Soften and flow!

All the ancient entrainments,
I now let you go.
Soften and flow,
Soften and flow!

All the wrongful decisions,
I now let you go.
Soften and flow,
Soften and flow!

All the terrible lies,

I now let you go.

Soften and flow,

Soften and flow!

All my stored up emotions

I now let you go,

Soften and flow,

Soften and flow!

This process is the most fun if you can allow ONE TO FLOW TO THE OTHER naturally as you naturally think of more things you'd like to let go of because they really have started to bug you, or you're so fed up with them, or you just simply want to get rid of them.

The alphabetical list that follows was generated in exactly that fashion, in a couple of afternoons.

If you want to, you can also:

- Work your way through the alphabetical list;
- Find some key words there to get going or for daily practice;
- To show someone else who needs a bit of a nudge to get the whole process started up;
- See the list as an example of how globally applicable this is, how wide reaching and simply pleasant and useful.

Take a look at this list now, from just three sessions with three different people. They are always surrounded by the spell form of:

All of my (...) I now let you go,

Soften and flow, soften and flow!

Abilities
Abuse
Abusers
Accidents
Accusations
Accusers
Achievements
Affectations
All that still hurts me
All that still scares me
All that still limits me
All that still blocks me
Ambitions
Ancient Entrainments
Angers
Answers
Anxieties
Allegiance/s
Allergies
Altruisms
Appraisals
Arrogance
Aspirations
Bad habits
Badness
Barriers
Barriers to (...)
Beliefs
Betrayals
Bindings
Blessings
Blocks to my magic
Blocks to the future
Boredom
Borders & Barriers
Bravery
Brutal criticisms
Burdens
Clownery
Clumsiness
Commands
Complaints
Conclusions
Connections

Constrictions
Contortions
Contracts
Controls
Courage
Cowardliness
Craziness
Crimes
Criticisms
Cruelties
Crutches
Curses
Damage
Damnation
Deceit
Defeats
Definitions
Delights
Delusions
Delusions of Grandeur
Demons
Depression/s
Descriptions
Desires
Despair
Desperation
Dilemmas
Dirtiness
Disappointments
Dislikes
Dissatisfaction
Distress
Divisions
Doubts
Dramas
Dreams
Duties
Ego/s
Enemies
Enslavements
Entrainments
Envy
Embarrassments
Emptiness

- Evil
- Excuses
- Expectations
- Errors
- Exhaustions
- Failure/s
- Fears
- Fears and Judgements
- Findings
- Fights
- Flirtations
- Flights of Fancy
- Fog
- Foggy Thinking
- Foolishness
- Foolhardiness
- Freedoms
- Friends
- Friends & Lovers
- Frozen energies
- Frustrations
- Games
- Genetics
- Ghosts
- Ghosts of the past
- Gifts
- Goals
- Good habits
- Goodness
- Gratitude
- Greed
- Gremlins
- Grief
- Grimness
- Guilt
- Guilty Feelings
- Habits
- Happiness
- Hatred
- Hopes
- Hungers
- Hurtful (...)
- Hurtful Decisions
- Ideas
- Ideas about (...)
- Ideas about people
- Ideas about me
- Illnesses
- Illusions
- Imaginings
- Injustice
- Insanities
- Interventions
- Irritations
- Instances of (...)
- Jealousys
- Jewels
- Joys
- Judgements
- Kindness
- Knowledge
- Laws
- Laziness
- Learnings
- Lies
- Lies and Deceit
- Life Lines
- Likes
- Limitations
- Logic
- Logical Fallacies
- Loneliness
- Longings
- Loves
- Madness
- Malcontent
- Maps
- Measures
- Memories
- Memories of injustice
- Memories of pain
- Mindgames
- Misery
- Mercy
- Merits
- Misplaced Allegiances
- Misplaced (...)
- Mistakes

Mistreatments
Monsters
Monstrosity
Morals
Morals and Values
Naivety
Niceness
Nightmares
Neediness
Negative Feelings
Obligations
Old wife's Tales
Opinions
Oppressions
Oppressors
Orders
Orders & Commands
Paranoia
Parts
Patience
Perturbances
Perversions
Pictures
Pictures of (...)
Pity
Plans
Plans & Goals
Positive Feelings
Possessions
Post Hypnotic Suggestions
Powers
Powergames
Prisons
Problems
Problems with (...)
Promises
Prejudices
Pretensions
Pretend (...)
Prides
Procrastinations
Punishment
Questions
Racial Burdens
Rage
Rat Races
Reality
Real (...)
Responsibilities
Restrictions
Reticence
Revenge
Revenge Fantasies
Reversals
Rewards
Righteous Indignation
Romantic Delusions
Routine/s
Scales
Sensations
Sensible Solutions
Sensitivity
Self Pity
Self Mutilations
Self Love
Self Hatred
Self Destruction
Self Satisfaction
Self Doubt
Separations
Salvations
Shields
Shocks
Shadows
Shoulds
Shyness
Snide Comments
Silences
Silliness
Sins
Skills
Slave Mentality
Slavery
Solutions
Sounds
Soulful Sighs
Stoppers
Stored Up Resources

Stress
Stressors
Superstitions
Stubbornness
Stupidity
Suffering
Surrenders
Suspicions
Talents
Tensions
Ties
Ties to (...)
Tiredness
Tired Old Games
Toys
Torments
Tormentors
Tortures
Torturers
Traumas
Trainings
Triumphs
Trust
Truths
Ugliness
Unfounded (...)
Unfounded Accusations
Unfulfilled (...)
Unfulfilled Desires
Unhelpful Orders
Unreasonable Nonsense
Untruths
Vanity
Victories
Views
Violence
Voices
Vows
Walls
Wants
Wars
Waterloos
Weakness
Weariness

Wild Accusations
Wisdom
Wishes
Words
Works
Worries
Wounds
Wrongful Decisions
Years
Yearnings

Comments On The Freedom Spells

The Power Of Releasing The Positives

It has been my experience that we seem to have no idea at all what we're doing here with these incarnations, and that just about everything we've ever thought we understood, worked out or believe is either just some total madness or delusion, or otherwise highly suspect and can't be relied on to produce a BETTER TOMORROW than all the yesterdays have proven themselves very practically to have been.

Therefore, this list doesn't only have "rage and sorrow" on it, but also things like joy, delight, holiness and their likes.

I propose that if we still think in terms of getting an A in a maths class as a "personal triumph", we very practically limit our own endeavours, and kill our futures in the process.

It is best to let all of that go, including things which felt so wonderful at the time, because that really clears the decks and makes room for NEW AND OTHER EXPERIENCES TO FINALLY GET A CHANCE TO MANIFEST.

The Guiding Stars breakthrough was that "good" or even "wonderful" stuff limits incarnations more powerfully than the greatest traumas ever could; abused children only turn into paedophiles and rapists themselves if there was a POSITIVE GUIDING STAR COMPONENT to the experience and never otherwise.

We might not be either by the grace of God, but that doesn't mean that we don't have our own versions of such truly terrifying misconnections lurking in our neurologies and energy systems which faithfully try to get us "the best there is" in every way.

Letting go of the positives may prove to be more freeing than the cessation of pain and fear that people so often think would give them salvation.

Releasing Questions

One of the core processes by which we drive ourselves structurally and very practically into an early grave is the question of questions.

I refuse to answer questions on EmoTrance, for example, if they are posited by people who know nothing about EmoTrance, because such questions are totally unanswerable and lead to insanity in every way.

Someone who hasn't a clue how ET works comes along and writes to the list, "If you do EmoTrance, and the client's head falls off, what do you do THEN?"

As you can see, it really is pointless even TRYING TO ANSWER THAT because the question itself is based on all sorts of bizarre assumptions that have absolutely nothing to do with reality and thus, can only lead into further delusion and madness if I even tried to answer that.

This is the trouble with most of our worst questions, speaking as a human here for a moment, in exactly the same structural way.

"If you have been bad and you die and go to hell, do you then ..."

That's the same as asking what you should do if someone's head falls off during an ET session. IF that person had ANY IDEA of the TRUE REALITY of an ET session, this question could not possibly be asked at all and indeed, it SHOULD NOT BE ASKED FROM SUCH A PLACE OF UNKNOWINGNESS ABOUT ABSOLUTELY EVERYTHING.

I propose that we are better off NOT ASKING any longer about things we have no experience of, or totally the wrong end of the stick in our delusions, such as, "Who am I?" or, "Does God exist?" or, "How do I get to be a better person?"

Soften and flow, let those questions go ...

... and you never know, you might then learn to come up with some REAL questions that can REALLY be answered by logic and observation of reality itself, and then ...

... we're getting somewhere!

Shedding The Stored Up Fat ....

Ah I enjoyed that heading.

Getting rid of old goals and plans, decisions, labels, responsibilities, values, and morals is such a wonderfully freeing experience, one can really feel oneself getting LIGHTER as one does that, EASIER, and in the right direction.

Don't be afraid to get rid of your morals, your ideas of kindness, mercy or compassion.

ALL OUR HUMAN IDEAS of these things are highly suspect and only if we get rid of the false labels and cross currents do we have any chance whatsoever to discover our true morality, our own very personal true experiences of what mercy or compassion actually really are.

I've had one or two experiences with that kind of thing and it has never failed to totally blow me away just how inordinately BETTER, STRONGER, RIGHTER AND MORE AMAZING IN EVERY WAY the new direct experiences were than what I'd been told was the meaning of service, love or responsibility.

Favourite Hangers On

And yes, I do think that the ones that you want to let go of the least are the ones that will do us all the most good in every way.

Letting go of evil is easy but can you let go of being good honest white lighter?

And yet I know you already know deep down that if you did, you'd get your chance to really become the real thing, not an impostor or someone who's forever TRYING to be that.

I propose that our totalities KNOW that what we THINK is a good white lighter IS A MILLION MILES OFF THE MARK and by chasing after the illusion or delusion endlessly, we are poodling down the wrong karmic path and making a major mess of our timelines.

So.

Over to you.

Start somewhere and let this "Freedom Spell" turn into a torrent of desire for more freedom, more release, more energy now finally flowing freely.

This doesn't just feel good.

It leaves your mind with a dawning appreciation of what we can do if we start to think logically and deal with true reality.

Have fun as always,

I certainly did!

Silvia Hartmann

November 2004

PS - A Brief Note On Using Freedom Spells With Clients

The standard schools of psychology hold it that we need to talk people out of their ideas that they are weasely, useless, miserable, stupid, insane idiots that don't even deserve to be spat upon.

You can use the Freedom Spell to for once give folk the chance to get to town and make a really honest list of all their shortcomings – and then let it all go, one after the other.

All of my weakness, I now let you go ...

All of my self destructiveness, I now let you go ...

All of my dumbness, I now let you go ...

In that way, finally their personal experiences and feelings are properly acknowledged and validated in all their dire darkness as their real reality experience for once – and then, there's the way out as well. Next session, you can do the things they pride themselves on and when you've got rid of those, they're clearer and more holy than some guy with a full-on calling trying to become a priest after 4 years in the seminary trying to be humble. In essence, what you are then left with is pure potential and a glimpse of real freedom in an incarnation – and I would say that would be worth having.

BeauTy T – Healing The Shattered Body Image

Beauty T – A General Introduction

We have a body, an energy body, and thanks to our consciousnesses, also an AUTOGENIC BODY which represents the conscious map our MINDS have constructed over our entire lifetime.

This Autogenic Body interferes in the functioning of the energy system, and therefore, also in the functioning of the physical body.

In most people, the Autogenic Body is a FAULTY CONSTRUCT that seems to be much worse than it actually is.

This happens when someone is told that their breasts are not big enough, or too big, or that OTHER KINDS OF BREASTS are BETTER somehow.

You need to be TOLD this by someone or something to create a judgement rule in your autogenic body, and this someone who tells you this may very well be YOU.

Either way, as soon as "judgements" happen in the autogenic body, such as:

- My breasts are too small and that is the reason why I cannot find love, therefore I hate my breasts.

... severe disturbances occur in the energy system as a PART OF THE BODY BECOMES HATED AND REJECTED.

As soon as ANYTHING becomes hated and rejected, communication to that part is lost or disturbed, and these disturbances ripple out wider and wider, the longer the disconnection is in place.

These disturbances then manifest to a person in the form of EMOTIONAL DISTURBANCES, such as:

Sadness, anger, low energy, fear, anxiety, stress.

These EMOTIONAL DISTURBANCES now impact back on the consciousness and the THOUGHT SYSTEMS OF THE MIND, leading to disturbed logic and reasoning, which manifests in THOUGHTS AND IDEAS such as:

I'm unlovable.

I'm insane.

There's something terribly wrong with me.

I'm ugly.

Such thoughts now drive further emotions and finally behaviour, such as not going out at all, trying to hide offending parts, getting surgery and many others which are all missing the point.

You can only change that which you love.

If someone hates and mistreats a house plant, or any part thereof, such as the leaves or the roots, they will not ever get to see what THE REAL PLANT WOULD HAVE LOOKED LIKE if it had received better care and attention.

Likewise, we don't actually know yet what we would look like if we were our true selves and WE WOULD SEE OURSELVES PROPERLY rather than a completely distorted "self image" that was constructed out of random people's random comments, societal fashion images and a great deal of self mutilation.

Even if plastic surgery is for someone the desired outcome, we should put it to them that they should make an effort first to SEE THE REAL BODY before deciding to operate upon it.

BeauTy will help you see your own body, feel your own body, and help you come to a realistic idea of what you really are, how you really work, and at the end of day, what you really look like.

Only when we know THAT can we make REALISTIC CHANGES to anything at all.

Back To BeauTy Basics

In order to move past all the various ideas about your body you may have spent a lifetime collecting and worrying about, and get a realistic handle and a sound, solid base from which to start, we are going to simply return to some absolutely unarguably TRUE facts.

As most "ideas" about the way you look are only based "ON OPINIONS" and not on facts, facing these very basic truths about your body is a good starting point.

These are the facts, in brief.

1. You are here, you have a body.
2. This body was NOT made by your parents, because they wouldn't begin to know how to make something this complicated.
3. Instead, it came into being as the direct result of the work of the CREATIVE ORDER.
4. Your ancestry traces right back, generation upon generation back in time, long past the time of man, long past the time of man-like beings, long before the dinosaurs walked the Earth, long, long before any creature at all came into being, and way back further still, before the oceans were born, right back until the time the entire Universe came into being.
5. Thus you are very practically related to all and everything there is.
6. As all things which were created by, from and through the Creative Order are beautiful (of course!), so must your body be beautiful – as deeply structurally beautiful as any fish, any insect, any star in the sky and any cloud in the heavens, by ITS VERY NATURE.
7. Furthermore, the body is NOT a collection of separate bits which may be judged harshly to create nonsensical divisions, but it is in all truth, ONE SINGLE ORGANISM that flows and moves, it is ONE BODY.

These are the only things which are being affirmed and re-discovered during the BeauTy T process, and they are all true:

1. **We have one single body;**
2. **It was made by the Creative Order;**
3. **It is hard working to give us life;**
4. **And being made BY the Creative Order, it is BELOVED, and HOLY.**

These four simple ideas, delivered with volition and in the intensity of a direct communication, be it between a client and an ETP, or a single person delivering this to themselves in self help, WILL HEAL the ravages of the autogenic disturbances from the ground up and will further provide a BASE LINE of truth to which one may return again and again, if disturbances have put us off balance.

What is Beauty T?

Beauty T is a special session of 30 minutes which is given by an ETP to a client outside of ordinary treatments or counselling. It is a PREMIUM SERVICE that is entirely positive and uplifting, in fact Beauty T is what you might call some serious icing on any humans cake.

- When a new Beauty T practitioner first begins to offer this service, I recommend that they pick some of their favourite clients and offer a "Try Me!" treatment at a special offer price. This is for the practitioner to gain confidence and delight in conducting this unusual but so very wonderful treatment that is more of lifetime's experience than any kind of therapy.

The Process of Beauty T

Very simply put, the ETP spends five minutes of the 30 minute session in rapport with the client and briefly explaining the idea of the treatment.

For the next 20 minutes, the ETP will simply go over the clients entire body and affirming the beauty of any and all of their physicality.

This is intensely hypnotic and training in the suggestive aspects inherent in Beauty T will be given during the Beauty T Practitioner training.

As the ETP affirms the beauty of the physicality, they will also seek to dispel with their words, with their touch and with their attitude NEGATIVE ENERGIES THAT HAVE INFESTED the energy systems.

- **Beauty T thereby represents a form of totality massage whereby:**
- **The ETP addresses the conscious mind in words;**
- **The energy systems with their own energy and intention;**
- **And the physicality with their touch,**
- **... All at the same time to produce a heightened state of lucidity across the client's entire existence.**

This experience, even with a total novice ETP, is unlike anything the client has ever been given, or has ever received.

It is intensely emotional for both the client as well as for the ETP and the benefits are simply incalculable.

Here are just some of the benefits a client can confidently expect from a Beauty T treatment:

Benefits Of Beauty T For The Client

- Radically new and different viewpoint on their bodies and all their bodies functions and appearances;
- Reconnection of physical sensations, emotional energies and ANOTHER HUMAN BEING which represents a MILESTONE EXPERIENCE that for many people has been sadly lacking all their lives;
- Beginning of a deep, profound and immensely healing change in their AUTOGENIC BODY and thus, their own relationship to their own selves for the better;

- Form of deep energising, renewal and celebration of the self that leaves the client clearer and more balanced than they may ever have experienced before;
- Working towards acceptance and celebration, if not worship, of the CREATOR GIVEN PHYSICALITY IN ALL ITS UNFOLDMENTS is a radical departure from the general paradigm of "fault finding and fault removal".

Beauty T is the long missing antidote to feelings of dislike of the self, unworthiness, ugliness, and depression or anger. It really works like an injection of positivity, unconditional regard and indeed, beauty energy into our depleted systems and brings them back to life.

But there is more than just the client soaking up energies they have been sorely and desperately lacking their entire lives.

It is impossible to do Beauty T as a practitioner and not also to feel the benefits of calling in and handling positive and unconditional energies of admiration, regard, love and worship.

Giving is as powerful and perhaps more powerful still than the receiving.

We all have so much love inside of us, and so few opportunities in the rigid structures of our societies and in our own personal prisons of entrainment to let this flow out and through, for the practitioner this also is a way to become far more powerful with every application of this, with every practice on every client.

THE MORE BEAUTY T YOU DO WITH PEOPLE, THE MORE POWERFUL A HEALER YOU WILL BECOME.

It becomes easier and easier with just a little practice to step into that place of unconditional regard, and this is a REAL FEELING and a REAL EXPERIENCE, not some pretend "I see the light within" if there isn't yet any light to be seen, BECAUSE NO-ONE'S EVER BOTHERED TO LIGHT THAT PERSON'S CANDLE FLAME as yet.

Beauty T is addictive.

That is not a bad thing, but indeed a WONDERFUL state of affairs, and not just for the practitioners who can't help but want to do this more, with a wider range of people, more profoundly and more deeply.

It is a wonderful thing for the client too, because they will seek the validation and REALITY CREATION of these new states of being.

When someone comes along and looks at this client and thinks or says, "Ooh you're so old, fat and ugly," the client has now and for the first time ever COUNTER EVIDENCE to fall back upon, and an answer to this – "I am as the creator made me. I am beautiful and I know this. How sad that you cannot appreciate this yet."

The client will begin to ACTIVELY SEEK OUT people who reflect this new order of being in their environment very practically – this is a practical AND an energetic effect, as perpetrators are magically attracted to the perpetual victims. One ceases to be a victim and the perpetrators stay away because there is nothing to feed on, nothing to stoke, nothing to be gained for them but defeat.

There is also absolutely no harm in a client who may have had a number of Beauty T sessions to return for more, after a break-up of a relationship say which left them vulnerable to the old self doubts, just the same as one would seek a headache pill for a headache, or a massage after a strenuous game of sport.

Beauty T Self Help

For both practitioners and clients and indeed any human being, the self help version whereby the person tells their own body directly how beautiful it is, how beloved by the creator itself, and how grateful they are for its services is a secondary device which brings the true power of Beauty T really into focus for long term.

I hold that it is too hard to expect from someone who has NEVER BEEN TOLD BY ANYONE that they are beloved and beautiful to pull themselves out of the swamp by their own hair. Especially if it has been said to be the wrong colour, thickness and texture and is entirely rejected ...

Make no mistakes.

Just as you can depress a child to the point of self mutilation by throwing endless hatred, negativity and fault finding at it, and then beyond into a state of dumb suffering where suffering is all there is and indeed all attempts at life have stopped, you can do this to your very own body, body parts, and many of us have done that too.

Renewal and healing cannot progress under such desperate circumstances.

The parts must be brought back to life, back into the light and ONLY non-conditional acceptance and positivity can EVER accomplish this.

This is the first Sleeping Beauty kiss to wake up parts of us, all of us, and once awoken even ever so slightly, these parts will begin to operate differently.

FIRST, THE CHANGE OF ATTITUDE.

THEN, THE INCREASING BENEFITS OF MANIFESTING CHANGE.

That's how it works, and it can't work any other way.

You cannot grow a good plant by withholding water, and you cannot grow a beautiful and flexible body by withholding love, admiration, support and the cheers of a victory parade to make it work extra hard for you.

Beauty T self help treatments come AFTER the practitioner has broken the ice and turned around a self destructive system of mechanisms that have caused so many problems over so many years.

This is one of the times when the inherent POWER AND AUTHORITY of the healer may be used to its full effect.

People have come to you for help.

They respect you and accept you as an authority.

WHEN YOU SAY THEY ARE BEAUTIFUL AND YOU MEAN IT, THEY CAN BEGIN TO ACCEPT THIS AND LEARN THAT IT IS TRUE.

The Client Practitioner Dance

The true hallmark of EmoTrance is the dance between the practitioner and the client, the fact that both work together and both gain immeasurably from this cooperation.

They gain different things in different ways, but both gain from the dance of giving and receiving.

For a practitioner who may have issues with their own nose, the challenge of reaching for and FINDING that reality where someone else's nose is indeed, creator given and because of that, simply beautiful is intensely healing in its own right.

Their own prejudices and disturbances sigh with pleasure and resolve at the same time; or at least are so challenged by this NEW INFORMATION, these NEW EXPERIENCES that they can no longer run their automatic self destructive spirals as once they did.

If this is done wholeheartedly then the world does become a different place as we are retraining ourselves to see the beauty and perfection in all things, and strive to encourage that beauty and perfection in its attempts to flower and unfold, wherever we see it, wherever we find it.

That is the Even Flow, and that is a truly holy thing to be doing.

I believe it is the core and the key of all true spirituality.

The challenge of finding this love and adoration for the physicality of other humans is profound and the rewards are equally profound in every way.

Beauty T is the first of a whole new breed of energetic healing strategies, one that works ONLY with the power of joy and the beauty of the creative order, and makes EXACTLY THAT AND ONLY THAT the antidote to the existing suffering.

The more damaged something is, the more unhappy it is in appearance or expression, the more love and unconditional regard it needs to be restored to its rightful functioning.

It is very simple really.

Frighteningly simple.

Now all we have to do for ourselves and for each other is to TRY OUR BEST to make it happen.

Wholeheartedly means simply that we give everything we have.

If that everything isn't very much, it doesn't matter because it is ALL THERE IS AND WE HELD NOTHING BACK.

It is the best we could do and every time we do it, we deserve a medal.

And we do get it, in the form of results and new feelings for ourselves, new and better and simply DIFFERENT experiences than we were led to believe were even available to us as human beings.

Beauty T As A Major Benefit For EmoTrance Clients

As usual, Beauty T could not even have arisen if it wasn't for EMOTRANCE FIRST.

To be able to accept the beauty of something that one has hated and blamed for one's entire life's problems for many years (such as the hair, the nose, the weight, the cellulite, the sex organs et al) one needs to do major energetic and emotional as well as neurological repair work.

One needs to be able to understand that the nose is not the problem, but the injuries pertaining to the AUTOGENIC NOSE and all the decisions and ideas and bad experiences that have cascaded since then from that injury (or those many injuries, as these things become self affirming and more and more real seeming over time, and of course, ever more painful and hurtful).

For clients with major well defined "body image problems" it is therefore essential that they are either treated for those specific problems up front and the energetic contortions that exist are cleared up BEFORE a full Beauty T treatment is even a possibility, OR that they are able to DO EMOTRANCE well and in the field already to do their part on the other end, that of being able to receive the incoming information/sensation packages from the ETP.

Beauty T PinPoint

You can therefore offer special Beauty T pinpoint sessions that deal with "the fat", or "the ears", or, "the hair" before a full Beauty T session becomes the first goal to have reached in the treatment flow and progression.

More than one such pin point session may be scheduled, and you can treat this entirely as a plastic surgeon would – start with the "worst parts" and work your way through in consultation with the client until they are ABSOLUTELY PERFECT IN EVERY WAY – at which point the real Beauty T treatments of total re-unification into ONE BEAUTIFUL TOTALITY may begin.

This is truly a breakthrough set of treatments and strategies that will produce so many benefits to both the clients as well as the ETPs, the potential is breathtaking.

With every client YOU TREAT and thereby STOPPING THEM FROM GOING TO A PLASTIC SURGEON, you are SAVING LIVES IN THE LONG TERM.

Plastic surgery has severe and mostly unacknowledged long term consequences. People in their desperation don't understand that in 30 years from now, the scar tissue formed back then is going to cut their lives short and lead to so much pain and suffering that they wish they'd never undertaken this.

You are bringing years of optimal functioning and the possibilities of that to your clients. And indeed, your clients will easily understand this once they are able to look beyond the length of their own nose, it being no longer a big autogenic issue that blocks their view of real and true reality after your treatments of them.

As to increased joy, libido, sense of lightness and pro-activity, better energy, better digestion, less risk of addictions, heart attacks and so much more, Beauty T is the perfect tool for a world that has gone insane with the quest for Beauty with the knife.

Beauty T is an enormously powerful concept.

It is incredibly easy to sell because those on the quest for Beauty will "try everything".

If they try THIS, and you get it right as the practitioner, they will have finally found what they have been looking for – a beauty that no age can take away, something that will be with you until your dying day, and that actually FEEDS AND SUSTAINS ALL YOUR FUNCTIONINGS, from mental clarity to physical recovery and immune system functioning.

The desperate quest for beauty is here, and we have with Beauty T a product that is not only fantastically holistic, but also DESPERATELY NEEDED BY MILLIONS.

It is safe.

It is a completely new and entirely surprising experience.

It works.

It heals, it helps and it uplifts.

It is self sustaining and NOT tied to the practitioner.

It is **a healing star** that passes right into the client's own hands as soon as they are ready and THEY IN TURN MAY AND WILL PASS IT TO OTHERS IN THEIR PATH.

Charging For Beauty T

You can do what you like with it.

You can pick your target audience and set to work – teenage girls, rich middle-class bored women, models who have just turned 23, football players. Anyone and everyone. You can advertise it for "long term weight loss". You can keep it as a premium service for your best EmoTrance clients.

You can run groups, workshops, retreats based around a progression of pinpoint Beauty T and the whole spectrum treatments.

You can charge what you like for a set of 21 sessions, or for one, or for ten or three – please remember that a breast reduction or a "tummy tuck" cost thousands of pounds and carries a penalty of long term health and psychological problems in its wake.

You can save your clients years of suffering and thousands upon thousands on quick fix or quack services and solutions, so charge what you want to charge for this, and if you don't want to charge anything at all, then don't.

I'd love to see at least some of you advertising along the lines of, "Thinking of Plastic Surgery? Try Beauty T First! First treatment at a special offer price!"

BeauTy T – Example Wording

Here is a transcript of the BeauTy T session I recorded for self help. These are in essence the words involved and the progression of neuro-energetic events which create the RECONNECTION between the mind and the autogenic body, in love and appreciation.

Find yourself comfortable and at ease.

Sit down, lie down,

And simply relax for a moment.

I am not asking you

To believe what I say today,

Just that you listen,

That you listen

And that you hear

The words I say.

As you are breathing ocean tides,

In and out, calmly and regularly,

And as you're becoming aware

Of your brave lionheart that beats,

And beats, and brings you life
And strength and endeavour,
You can become aware
Of your entire body,
A beautiful creation, always in flow,
Connected to the deepest realms
Given to you by the Creative Order itself.
Your relatives are the stars in the sky,
The grey mountains, the green vales,
The deepest oceans.

You are, as they are,
Children of the Universe.

And now, I would speak to you
About your beautiful hands,
About your beautiful, flexible,
Hard working hands,
That may draw symbols,
Carry loads,
That may stroke your own skin,
Touching and receiving both,
Your beautiful, perfect hands,
Beloved.

Your beautiful perfect fingers
And your hands and your wrists,
Flexible and yet so strong,
And the skin above,
Sensitive to the finest touch,
The slightest breath of wind,
Your strong, beautiful arms,
Your flexible elbows,
Beloved all,
All a part of this, your body.
Stroke your arms
With your mind
And express your gratitude,
For all the hard work,
All those years,
Beautiful.

Beautiful you are,
Your strong arms,
And your strong,
Strong shoulders and your back,
Your powerfully flowing spine,
All the way up across your back,
Carrying the most essential messages,
Flowing all the time,
Every day,

In absolute perfection,
Beloved, beautiful spine,
Strong powerful,
All the way up
To your strong, strong neck,
That lovingly holds your head,
Flexibly, all directions,
All dimensions,

And there is your hair,
Beautiful, as the creator has given it to you,
Of the self same structure
As the stars in the sky,
With loving hands and loving gratitude,
Stroke your hair all the way down
To your neck and shoulders.

And there is your beautiful face,
Perfect forehead, perfect skin,
Exactly in flow, as the creator wanted it to be,
Perfect protection, perfect love.

Your eyebrows and then your lids,

And your beautiful eyes

Which do not only let you

To see the world,

But in return,

Allow you to touch

Those things you give attention to -

With your stroking attention of love

You nourish those things

That are around you.

And then there is

Your perfect nose,

Perfect in all ways

Just as the creator designed it to be,

Your cheek, your jaw,

Powerful and strong,

Ever working for you,

Ever working hard,

Your perfect lips

That shape the words you speak

And give the kiss of love

To those things

You most admire.

Your chin
And then your perfect neck and throat,
Your voice,
Gently sliding down across the one body,
Towards your beautiful, strong chest,
Where your brave lionheart beats
With such regularity, with such power
And with such ease,
Where your breath is the tide of life,
Flowing through and out,
Always, always, beloved celebration
Of taking in
The life from the universe,
And releasing your contribution
In return.

Your beautiful breast,
Perfect, absolutely perfect as
Designed by the creator,
And oh so beloved,
And your strong powerful chest,
And your stomach, digestion moving
Keeping you alive,
Giving you the power
And the energy you need
To do your work here in this world,

To dance with joy here in this world,
Your beautiful, beloved stomach,
And your beautiful, perfect genitals,
Made by the creative order
That made the stars and the skies above,
The galaxies in all their glory,
And the sunrise too,
Perfectly beautiful,
Pure and incontrovertible,
Always, always,
And regardless of what the will of man
Might falsely think or do decree,
And then there are
Your powerful hips,
Flexible, strong,
And from your powerful hips
We may stroke lovingly across
Your wonderful buttocks,
Such powerful muscles beneath your skin,
So sensitive so perfect
And as beloved as
Your strong and powerful thighs,
Strong straight bones,
And your wonderful,
Flexible knees that lightly move
With every thought, with every breath,

As we slide lightly and with admiration
Down towards your calves and ankles,
Your flexible ankles
That keep your balance
Regardless of what
Other things you might find,
Or whether you go up a steep incline,
Or down towards a perfect valley,
Your perfect ankles support you -
And then there are your trusty feet,
Oh so necessary and so deeply beloved.

Now feel a breath of wind, of life,
Touch you from your toes that slides
All the way across your body,
To your hair and out,
And hear it,
Feel it,
Know it:

> Your body,
>
> ONE BODY,
>
> Your beautiful body,
>
> Given to you by the Creator,
>
> Your beautiful body,
>
> Always in flow,
>
> Always beloved
>
> And BEAUTIFUL.
>
> *BeauTy T Self Help Transcript 2004*

BeauTy T - In Conclusion

Beauty T is truly new and revolutionary in its concept.

It is in full keeping with ALL true spiritual traditions and celebrates the Creative in every way.

It is completely positive and totally healing in its application, and it is simple to do.

We have the tools and we have the experience to make it work, and to make a real change to the people who we treat with Beauty T, as well as to ourselves.

Please let us not waste this opportunity to do some REAL GOOD, and make a LASTING DIFFERENCE not just to ourselves and our clients, but by example, to everyone we come into contact with.

Beloved be,

Silvia Hartmann

April 2004

BeauTy T For Animals

All animals are extremely sensitive to all forms of energy occurrences. Further, as they cannot lie, when one applies energy healing or energetically based change work with animals, the results are clean, powerful and a total eye opener to those who are still not quite sure that yes, there is an energetic continuum, and yes, we can make REAL changes when we work in those realms.

BeauTy T, an EmoTrance Level 2 techniques set, is about love and attention to heal all manner of injuries in the energy system. It is amazing to do with people, but it's just as amazing when we apply it to animals, and especially beloved companions.

Here is a full protocol so you can try BeauTy T with your companion too!

BeauTy T For Animals

Earlier this year I conducted an advanced EmoTrance seminar called BeauTy T for people.

The core idea is for people who would go to a plastic surgeon because they hate a part of their bodies so much, to CHANGE THAT part of the body and their relationship with it using this "magical alternative".

In order for something magical to work on a par or BETTER than actual plastic surgery, it had to get pretty heavy duty, as you can imagine; those sort of disturbances for people are so dramatic, you need something very powerful to take it on, and it really needs to work and to be seen that it works.

When I got home from the seminar, I was pretty buzzy and later in the evening, I saw that my old dog needed exactly THAT thing we'd been doing all day with people, and I did it with the dog. It was very moving, so INCREDIBLY MUCH simpler than doing it with a person, and the old dog just blossomed in front of my eyes. My rather tearful eyes, at that, so also it changed MY attitude to the dog in the process.

As it is so very much simpler to do it with animals I thought I'd write up the basics of the process for you so you can have a go at BeauTy T with animals and experience the power of this remarkable process – and its very REAL results.

1. The Ambassador From The Creative Order

In order to make it work and get yourself in the right state for this, you CANNOT BE your normal self. You have to step into a different state of being and we practised this by saying up front, "Good morning, my name is Silvia and I stand before you today as A REPRESENTATIVE OF THE CREATIVE ORDER."

You need to try this a few times until you can really mean it and get a feel of this, if necessary tap on reservations or bad feelings in the body until it all flows smoothly.

2. The Truth About The Matter

Now, look at the animal, not as you but as the said representative of the creative order, and simply become aware that we are confronted with a SYSTEM THAT WAS MADE BY THE CREATIVE ORDER, directly, the same as the stars in the skies and mountains, clouds, ants and sunsets.

As such it is BEYOND ALL REPROACH, BEYOND ALL JUDGEMENT and AWESOMELY INCREDIBLE.

Completely regardless of what has happened to this creature, it is an example of the functional design, a work of art made by the Creator itself, doing the very best it can and doing this most fantastically.

That is THE TRUTH in all ways, about any creature, any manifestation; and even though you might like to try and hurt a creature, or poison an ocean, fell a tree, you could never ever CORRUPT it - no system from the creative order can be corrupted BY MEN. Damaged, yes. Destroyed and defaced, yes. But never CORRUPTED. It always retains its original perfection, its innocence - and its BEAUTY.

3. Delivering The Energy

Now, and no sooner than we have seen that BEAUTY that exists in every system the Creative Order designed, we tell the creature, reflect that beauty back at them, because it is THIS which heals so many people inflicted ravages of judgement, pain, insecurity.

With an animal, we do this simply by going from snout to tail, touching if possible, and saying, "You have a perfect nose, perfect teeth, perfect head and perfect ears. You are beautiful, and you ARE BELOVED."

Work your way all the way across the creature - perfect feet, made by the creative order so that you can walk, perfect, beloved - until the entire animal has been covered.

That can be moving, but it can also be funny - "Perfect beak, perfect feathers" can make you laugh and smile and that's a GOOD THING.

4. A Blessing To Complete

The last thing we do, after "your perfect tail" , is to straighten up, draw back the focus so you can encompass the entire creature, hold out your hands to it and say/send an overall blessing along the lines of, "One body, one perfect body, one perfect creature."

I'd like to finish up by saying that you can also do it just as a bye the bye, so rather than the full ritual, to just pat the creature on the head and think, "Perfect head, perfect intelligence, designed by the creative order ..." in passing, or at any time at all.

But to really get the hang of WHAT THAT IS, and HOW THAT FEELS when you even try it for the first time, I recommend trying a whole treatment with an animal that needs it.

They probably all do, they've all been judged and mistreated as we all have been, just as a side effect of living in these strange conditions as we and the creatures now do, so ...

BeauTy is a very powerful thing for change, for those who do it and those who receive it just the same.

It's not that difficult either and I think that by doing it with animals first, it is a lot easier all around; we have far less barriers to really getting our heads around the truth of these very basic things that then allow for really amazing and powerful energy healing experiences.

Energy Magic:
Creating A Powerful Training Ritual

A good ritual isn't something you copy out of a book, but something that feels right to all parts of you - that is when the planes come into alignment and it makes the correct conditions for very powerful magic and reality creation.

Rituals consist of components that an individual magician has assigned for certain purposes. Even when there are so called schools of magic, and everyone does the same ritual and has done it for millennia, there was still and always one individual magician at the bottom of it all, and that is worth remembering.

The more you yourself are exactly the same as that old magician, the more the ritual will fit, just as though you were wearing that person's actual robe, hat and shoes.

As magicians get along in their works and explorations, their alphabet of physical and non-physical symbols, such as chalices and demons, whatever, grows, and thus they get to create for themselves ever more complex (and complicated) rituals and routines. That is how you end up with great big ceremonies that have dozens of components, props and bits, words, actions, clothes, and all sorts.

To start out right, all we have to do is to each consider the following about a spell.

- Firstly, what is the core of that spell? Let's say beauty, for an example. When you start out with spells, make them simple and very cohesive, one topic, one desire, one outcome, like a laser light that is so powerful because all the frequencies are pure and the same.
- When you have that core, you can then assign objects which are resonant or the same TO YOU as this core thing. In our case, that would be beauty.

Now, in order to involve the totality, find:
1. Something you can touch, that when you touch it, you know it is BEAUTY for you. This may be a crystal (too cold for me

personally) or a silk scarf. It may even be a cat! The important thing is that now you have something that is IN ALIGNMENT with the core of the spell, and that being so, will strengthen it with its presence and by bringing in your physical touch and your physicality.

2. Something you can see, that when you see it, you know it is BEAUTY. I might pick the image of a plant, or animal, or a person, you on the other hand might pick a sunset or an ocean. It is idiosyncratic (specific to any one given person) and not transferable, as so many things in magic.

3. Pick something you can hear and when you hear it, you know that is BEAUTY. Music, natural sounds, someone's voice specifically, a particular tone on a particular instrument - whatever is correct for you, is correct.

4. Pick something that you can smell and when you smell it, you know that is BEAUTY. Perfume, incense or better still, the scent of something directly which can be much more powerful in every way than pre-processed or bottled things, such as a real lemon, or a real flower, or a spice or herb, or a cloth with somebody or some things scent on it.

5. Pick something you can taste, and when you taste it, you know that is BEAUTY. Try different things because to translate what we often first thought of as a strictly visual concept, like beauty, or a different idea, such as money or power, needs to be translated into this very powerful modality before eating beauty or money too is online and understood.

In the very act of assembling these objects and trying them out for yourself, rather than taking an "off the shelf" ritual that could have all the wrong meanings, energies and connotations for YOU PERSONALLY, you will already learn amazing things about the core request of your spell, even without having waved any magic wands just the once.

But now also, you are beginning to build up a multi-dimensional alphabet for creating a powerful ritual because these "beauty components" of course can be used again later and in combination with other core components, to create more elegant or complex magical events.

Let us turn now to the other aspects of the ritual.

Order & Sequence In The Ritual

A good ritual must have an order and sequence, a beginning, a middle and an end.

Now here again, the FLOW of the ritual, i.e. what you say, do, experience and eventually call into being, is personal and always once again, custom made to the core of the spell being cast.

With your five basic physical items present, now arrange them IN THE CORRECT ORDER AND SEQUENCE.

In our example, we have one particular magician who has picked:

To touch: A silk scarf

To see: A rose

To hear: Vivaldi Violin Concerto

To smell: Frankincense

To taste: Lemon

As you can clearly understand on all levels, this is HIGHLY IDEOSYNCRATIC and please know that I neither recommend any of these items, nor even would think to use them myself, as this is just an example.

Now, we simply ask ourselves, which one should be first?

An arrangement tends to appear quite naturally, and if it does not, we try it out and wait for the "cold, warm, hotter, YES!" click when we just know that something is right with every fibre of our being.

In this case, the person found this arrangement to suit them perfectly:

First, the music. Then, the scent. Then the scarf, then the taste, then look at the rose.

Now, and now that we have in all ways grounded ourselves physically in the reality of BEAUTY as it is perceived by our five human senses, we move along and into the magical, and from this groundswell of connection to the meaning of beauty, we stand up and we speak the spell.

Free Talismans

The interesting thing is that of course all the items that have been assigned to BEAUTY have now become free Talismans and powerful reminders, evocations and generally strengtheners of the spell, purely by being involved in the first place and without any major effort.

Later on, we get to make symbols of such events that encompass for example BEAUTY through all the planes in every way, but that's not yet and not even necessary.

The Talismans, even when nothing further is ever done, will retain a reminder and a remembrance of the spell and the intentions, wherever they appear and whatever the circumstance.

That and the building symbol library is of course a fascinating process in and of itself, as you will find out, and as you move forward with your own personal explorations and learnings.

The Ritual Surround

The basic 5 senses, gathering the energy, and then speaking the spell, process is now the core of the ritual itself.

Soon enough, magicians found out that regardless of the spell or the purpose of the spell, it is always useful to have a good entry point to the whole endeavour and a neat exit as well.

So they made a variety of rituals for THAT purpose, such as retreating to special places, casting circles, dancing about for a time, drumming to get into a "deep state of meditation" and so forth.

I hold that making such a big deal of the act of casting a simple spell, be it for luck in war or protection on travel, finding a new lover and so forth creates A DANGEROUS DIVIDE between the hard and the truth of reality.

It puts magical endeavours into this "special only on Sundays or if all else has failed" category, takes it OUT of our lives and that's not how it should be.

Our lives should be magical in all ways, all the time, every day, every night, and the lessons of true magic as well as our growing experience and power with these systems MUST BE A PART OF LIFE ITSELF.

Look. You are stuck at the side of a motorway because you've run out of petrol. It is raining, the middle of the night and you're tired.

You don't have any "ritual gear" in the trunk of your car nor the "meditation drums", nor even feel up to sitting there on a mat for two hours, trying to get yourself into a deep meditative state.

That is COMPLETELY USELESS for normal everyday life.

And it is important to note that these rituals you build for yourself become entrenched very quickly, and then there's no luck to be had anymore when the rabbits foot has been unfortunately lost.

That is NOT our kind of magic at all, so bearing this in mind, I suggest you:

1. Find an entrance and exit ritual for now that is extremely fast, extremely simple and does NOT require any form of external help, i.e. so that you can perform it in a prison cell, naked, and with nothing whatsoever to hand.

2. That you make sure, especially at the beginning, to lay all thoughts of previous notions and learnings as to "how difficult it is" to get that shift into the magical operations state, completely aside and simply shift into it, quickly, instantly, and most importantly, WITHOUT A FUSS.

Here are some examples of entrance and exit "rituals" to try or to give you an idea what you might do to make that shift as a beginner.

Imagine a strong image, such as the sun rising, for entrance into the ritual, and another, such as the sun being right above you in the sky for exit.

Say a word out loud or in your head, such as "Sunrise" for entry and "Day" for exit.

Click your fingers and get going, click them again when you're done.

Take three deep breaths in through the nose and out through the mouth for entry and exit.

Wriggle your nose!

Was that last one a joke?

Yes and no. Let's remember that magic is light as a feather, never dour and heavy, joyful and playful, and it cannot be approached in any other way, or you'll break its true spirit and get very little co-operation in return.

A First True Magical Ritual

Now, let's put our first ritual all together.

Ritual entrance:

One deep breath in through the nose, out through the mouth.

Energy gathering:

Put on the music, light the frankincense stick. Stroke the scarf, taste the lemon, now stand up and cast the spell:

Beauty comes to me

Beauty lives in me

Beauty I can see

It belongs to me.

Beauty is mine now,

Joyous and free,

This is my will,

And so shall it be.

Let the power of the spell resonate and when it is done,

Ritual exit:

One deep breath in through the nose and out through the mouth. All done!

The Rituals Exercise

Pick an essence such as Beauty that you would align yourself to and make friends with, and create your own magical ritual.

Conduct the ritual, and write down what you have learned.

Now, do the same with 6 more essences, always making notes of your experiences.

Lastly, look across the completed series of the 7 exercises and write down specifically what you have learned about the PROCESS OF ESSENCE RITUAL CREATION.

Magic Words

We had a meeting tonight to discuss some form of advertising strategy for In Serein 1.

After not getting anywhere at all for some time eventually I remembered a Nightingale Conant course I've had for many years called "Magic Words That Make Your Business Grow".

In essence the author says that if you can get the right words you can sell anything to anyone, and that the magic words are very specific and unique.

I'd never considered that energetically because this sort of thing was of course way way before Project Energy or such, but it is of course true that words can be "energetic containers", like attractive little blue perfume bottles that sparkle in the sunlight, to attract attention.

IS itself is completely peppered with powerwords. It is MADE UP of sequences of power words.

Here's just one single, random paragraph:

I caught him from the spiral of anger and despair and steadied him for a moment which was enough for him to regain control and push me away. The link snapped and he reached across me, shut the book with such force that the table creaked and moved.

Spiral. Anger. Despair. Control. Force.

Those things are the ubiquitous "power words".

If any one of those five words are IN THE HEADLINE of an advertisement, or a newspaper article, they attract "attention" because they **FLARE MORE BRIGHTLY** than less highly charged counterparts, such as "Mayor's Wife Opens Supermarket This Tuesday".

Once we got that, and it's actually very easy indeed, we made a list of major power words that turn up in In Serein over, and over, and over again because that would be the predominant energy flares that really are in that book, and those who would be attracted to THOSE VERY WORDS and find a resonance, would be actually the CORRECT

TARGET AUDIENCE for In Serein - and could get it from a few words, a headline, a short ad.

The energetic reality FLARES like a beacon or a lighthouse.

Isn't that fascinating?

Here are a few of the key "magic words" from In Serein.

- Power
- Logic
- Magic
- Love
- Justice
- Evil
- Beauty
- Violence
- Redemption
- Clarity.

Those are just a few from a list which also contains some adjectives, such as sensuous, hypnotic, innocent, decadent, spell binding and colour blessed.

Really all that is necessary is then to take the essential power words and put them together in a paragraph and description to get a very POTENT description or ad copy or summary or whatever going that really does cover the ESSENCE of the story/book but without having to get into too much detail or giving the whole game away.

But here's the deal.

When someone tries this who doesn't have a clue as to how to read the real existing energetic realities beneath the surface of the words themselves, OR uses power words that really do not pertain to the object in question (Blogbleach - The force of beauty solution magic for your toilet terrors) and just sticks them randomly end on end, you get a nasty uncomfortable mess.

I don't think we have this problem anymore. I really can't see (or feel) anyone here on this list who has done as much energy work as we have NOT being able to spot incongruencies in the flow of the ENERGY OF A HEADLINE OR ADVERTISEMENT USING POWER WORDS AND PHRASES.

Quick Power Words Exercises

Here are some quick energy magic exercises on our magic words.

- a) Spot power words for a few days in people's speech, on TV, in print ads.
- b) Check out your own products/services and find YOUR OWN MAGIC POWER WORDS YOU REALLY USE CONSTANTLY in the actual application of your work (ie WHAT you talk about rather than TALKING ABOUT IT).
- c) Start making some sentences out of those power words for soundbites, ads, your stationary, tag lines, short articles etc. and see if you can both retain the power of the words, and an EVEN FLOW of exactitude and correctness in describing what you're describing.

It's a basic energy magic strategy that will work on all and every form of advertising, right down to writing personal ads for dating agencies.

The Golden Line

The other day I was involved in a discussion about the concept of "The Golden Line" - a spiritual format of using the energies of people who went before us to help us NOW, support us from the other side.

Originally this would have been entirely ancestor based, but with one thing and another, it then went to a concept of "elders" who may or may not be genetically related, and from there to a more global concept of "teachers" which go on to form a timeline support group that reaches out into the past and continues with YOU being the next temporal member of the group.

Now as I have noticed recently, as one may have more than one single timeline, one can of course have more than one Golden Line.

There is no reason to not have both ancestral support, for example, as well as "teacher" support, and for modern folk such as ourselves I would propose a further version, namely that of the heroic golden line, or one composed of one's own personal heroes.

These would be people across time and space, real living people, not "sons of God" or suchlike (different form of Golden Line, different level), who have significantly contributed to our own incarnations, and most practically so.

For example, someone may have been significantly influenced by the teachings of Marcus Aurelius, or the life of the Yellow Emperor, or the writings of Shakespeare.

Everyone has these people, and as this is a highly energetic dimensional occurrence, it doesn't matter WHEN they were, or WHO they were. It doesn't matter WHY they had such an impact either - there are no brownie points in the impact department.

A young child that was tremendously moved by the simple kindness of an unknown person for ONE SECOND would be right to place such a person on their Golden Line, even if that person had never made it into the history books at all or was otherwise entirely unremarkable.

Or a pop singer, of whom everyone else said that they were stupid and puerile and worth nothing might have sang a song once which had an inordinate impact on a young person, or even an old one - it is the IMPACT that matters, not anything else.

From the moment of impact, the messenger (which is a better word than "teacher") exists as a connection in an individual's energy system, and they will remain there forever, as a TREMENDOUS resource, if only we know it.

Of course, with our own personal heroes we know this already.

We know what they did for us and how they CHANGED US. How valuable that was for us, and what the depth of gratitude is as a result we hold for them.

In the construction - conscious, volitionous construction! - of a Golden Line, we use the gratitude and awareness to deepen this connection, strengthen it and to USE it to HELP US NOW and in the future.

Peers & Repayments

You might be familiar with the term of "hero worship" which exists as a result of the initial impact the messenger had.

Of course, we worship them. They did something very, very special for us and further, they set US up to be able to do something like that eventually for others.

It's like an initiation into the general state of human heroes, the first step into a different unfoldment as a human being altogether.

Not everyone has heroes, and not everyone becomes eventually a hero to other people.

This is a very sad thing if you think about it, but there are also many steps and stages along the way which, if we are not consciously aware of them, will hinder the progress from star struck to becoming a star.

The Golden Line rituals take care of the most essential of these, and the first of them is what I've just said.

Namely that:

The outcome of the process that is initiated when someone becomes YOUR hero, is that YOU BECOME A HERO.

If we use the other term, the sentence above would read:

The outcome of the process that is initiated when someone comes to you as a MESSENGER is that you become a MESSENGER.

What keeps us stuck in the state of being the receiver of messages, rather than the bringer or broadcaster of messages, is the lack of RECIPROCAL REPAYMENT.

The Hero Transaction

There are certain laws in the universe and one of these is that taking and giving must be in a balanced flow situation so that systems function properly.

If this is not obeyed, you get very fat or very skinny people and all the problems which result from that, for just one practical example.

We feel immensely GRATEFUL to our own heroes and it is not UNTIL THIS HAS BEEN REPAYED do we become their PEERS - the energy exchange is then completed and a new system that can flow and GROW comes into being in that instant.

Now, here we once again are in an area where there is much planes confusion of old.

MATERIAL things CAN NOT repay a hero's debt.

You can build giant statues, cathedrals and pyramids until the end of days and the debt is not repaid in that way.

You can dedicate your life to become a priest to that person and worship at some altar every single day BUT THAT WILL NEVER REPAY THE DEBT.

The original transaction was a ONE TIME ENERGETIC EVENT and so the return transaction must be the same - it cannot be anything else or you are trading in the wrong currency.

A Unique Repayment

This one time energetic repayment for the hero's gift, which will in turn elevate us to their level and make a hero of ourselves in the giving of it, has to be highly personal both ways.

The champions dealings are strictly non-group based, they are intensely personal - from one individual human being to another, directly and no middlemen.

I am sure you have begun to give some thought as how you could possibly repay your hero.

Our ritual will have a number of components, but the first and foremost is that of acknowledging the champion and calling them by name.

1. Acknowledgement

Remember that all of this is ENERGETIC in nature and thus, needs no public advertisements or such (although you can, if you want to or desire to).

Pick a champion and begin to frame inside your mind a way of explaining how and why they helped you.

You can just think about this as you go for a walk or in meditation; a Project Sanctuary meeting where you can tell your champion exactly what they did for you and meant for you will serve most splendidly.

You can write a letter to this extent or give a talk about it, or just be clear inside yourself as to what it was that is being repaid.

This is setting the intensity and structure of energies that will also have to be involved in your counter-payment - there has to be balance at the end of the transaction so you can both be peers and clear of all ties and contortions.

2. The Champion's Gift

Now, we want to consider the individual your champion was or is, and what we might be able to give to them, uniquely and individually, that only we might give.

And this could be truly almost anything at all.

You might write a song for your champion, or create a special prayer; give them healing or a "The Gift"; create a Project Sanctuary habitat for them, give them interaction; you may plant a tree or shrub for them, pick a single flower or create a ritual of any kind.

Bear in mind that all physical actions or acting in accord is only there to strengthen the underlying ENERGETIC effects of what you are doing and not the end result or even purpose.

For example, if you choose to paint a special painting for your champion, it is not the painting that is the gift, but the ACT of painting it instead.

The simplest help I can give here to come up with the perfect contribution for your champion is just to sit and ask yourself, "What could I give this person to repay their gift to me so that we may both be raised and lifted and our exchange becomes complete?"

Something WILL come to you - all you have to do is follow it.

And that's as simple as that.

But being simple doesn't mean it isn't one of the most profoundly ADULT exercises for a human being to undertake.

One last comment I would like to make is to repeat that when a champion has been repaid and the transaction is complete, this does not at all mean that the relationship is over.

In the contrary.

It becomes a living relationship from that moment on; bright and new and a HUGE resource for both of you in every sense of the word.

It becomes a step stone for a whole new level of evolution and interaction, one that is both sublime and joyous, and a most wonderful experience.

Silvia Hartmann, 2004

EmoTrance – The Resolution

I have been aware of the existence of the energy universe consciously and absolutely since 1987, and the EmoTrance system, ostensibly for energy healing, energy consciousness and energy magic is my device to give others **a set of tools by which they can experience and evaluate these realities for themselves.**

The three levels of EmoTrance together create a bridge to the other side of my work, the other side of my research, and that is about human potential in general.

I have done my best with what I have to create a cohesive system with EmoTrance that serves above all as an invitation to experiment, to pay attention and to begin to work pro-actively with the endless manifestations of energetic occurrences in every day life.

The development of the ET usages, examples and techniques from 2002 to 2005 has been tremendously exciting and often surprising; the learnings and practical applications, from Thought Flow, to Heart Healing, Project Energy and Freedom Spells right up to the truly amazing Art Solutions process will continue to unfold, as they must.

I shall now go back to my original investigations into the least known and most mysterious aspects of the human energy system, the Psychic Circuitry or Astral Circuitry.

For this, it is essential to understand how we process and evaluate non-physical information, and that is the realms of metaphor as the interface device.

After the apprenticeship of EmoTrance, which taught us to come to energetic manifestations without prejudice and to LEARN about them, rather than to label and judge them, we can now go back to the essential angelic language that humans share, because it is the basic and deep structural process of reading the greater patterns of the Living Universe around us and becoming consciously aware of this, as is our birthright.

The next step on therefore is Project Sanctuary, and EmoTrance was always designed to be the structural and cognitive bridge to THAT.

I sincerely hope you have enjoyed the trip I chose to call EmoTrance as much as we all have, and I would like to take this opportunity to thank my co-researchers and co-developer Nicola Quinn, and also Steve Collins and Ananga Sivyer, who, like myself, do not do anything other than research and LIVING our theories in practice and all reality.

I thank you for your interest and I hope you have found something to excite you, inspire you and which will prove itself to be immensely USEFUL to you, more so as time goes by.

With all my best wishes,

Silvia Hartmann

May 19th, 2005

Addendum 2 - Further Information

About The Author

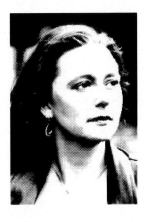

Silvia Hartmann PhD is a highly qualified and experienced trainer of Hypnosis, Hypnotherapy, Energy Therapies and Neuro-Linguistic Programming, author, international lecturer and motivational speaker. She is the Co-Founder and Director of The Association For Meridian & Energy Therapies and founder of the oldest established MET internet newsgroup, Meridian Therapy, as well as being a Contributing Editor to Gary Craig's EmoFree List.

With an extensive record in trainings design, she is well known for her outstanding ability to create trainings that allow the participants to understand and integrate even highly complex materials and making it easy to learn, easy to do and easy to replicate.

She is the author of numerous highly acclaimed original works in the field, including "Project Sanctuary" and "Guiding Stars 2002".

Silvia Hartmann's best-selling EFT Training Manual "Adventures In EFT" has to date been translated into four languages and is acknowledged to be "The Best Book on EFT".

After studying and re-searching Energy Psychology & Meridian Energy Therapies approaches in-depth for four years, Silvia Hartmann created EmoTrance™, a truly groundbreaking and entirely innovative approach to working with the human energy system for mental and physical health.

For Further Information about Silvia's Work please visit:

http://SilviaHartmann.com	Complete Online Catalogue of Manuals & Trainings
https://DragonRising.com	Books, Courses, Events, CDs etc.
http://EmoTrance.com	The Official EmoTrance Site, News, Events, Practitioner/Trainer listings & EmoTrance Shop

EmoTrance – Further Information
Oceans of Energy
The Patterns & Techniques of EmoTrance, Vol 1

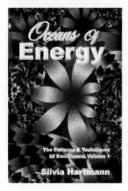

EmoTrance is a new system for handling the human energy body. 'Oceans of Energy' gives a thorough grounding in the underlying principles of EmoTrance™ for self help and use with others and introduces the uses of the system, namely self healing, healing others, goal setting, and state management, especially of new and previously un-experienced enlightenment states. Includes discussion of the developmental history of the system, stories from practitioners and first person reports of EmoTrance™ in the field.

Living Energy
The Patterns & Techniques Of EmoTrance, Vol 2

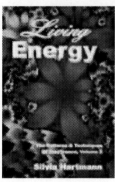

Living Energy, EmoTrance Vol. 2, concerns the extraordinary realities of the Autogenic Universe, the Thought Flow system, the HEROS systems and of Heart Healing.

This outstanding manual contains a full transcript of the first Living Energy presentation from 2003, plus many additional techniques, patterns and articles.

Become A Certified EmoTrance Practitioner – World Wide!

The Official EmoTrance Practitioner

Distance Learning Certification Training Course

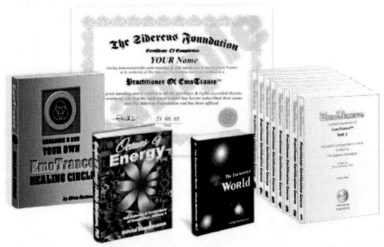

Study the extraordinary EmoTrance system of energy healing, spiritual healing and emotional healing in the comfort of your own home – anywhere in the world.

This exquisite, in-depth training, especially created for the distance learning student and containing a wealth of fantastic exercises, background information is certified by The Sidereus Foundation.

Upon successful completion, the new EmoTrance practitioner (ETP) will be able to join the growing international community of those who help others experience their worlds and themselves in a whole new way.

Reasonably priced, with full tutor support and many additional materials, this is an outstanding opportunity to bring the light and aliveness of EmoTrance to YOUR community.

The OFFICIAL EmoTrance Distance Learning Practitioner Course

Available from:

https://DragonRising.com

+44 (0)1323 729 666

Project Sanctuary

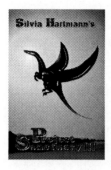

So now, we are working with the energy body, with thoughtfields, with meridians and energy shields and in the Quantum spaces where what we have learned about time, gravity, distance and more is no longer applicable. If we go into those spaces with our limited four-dimensional thinking, formed by the cause-and-effects of the physicality and after a lifetime of conditioning in the Hard, we will never be able to be at home here, never be able to actually understand and never mind affect these spaces and their processes as we should and as we can.

What is required is to learn a whole new way of thinking. A logic based on entirely different principles, on entirely different laws of nature – quantum logic. Project Sanctuary is probably the first training manual ever written in the history of humanity to be a self help guide and device to teach quantum logic and to make it easy for anyone who wishes to learn.

Fascinating from the start, utilising immediately what we have remaining by the way of connection to our intuition, creativity, magic and the wider realms of the universe, Project Sanctuary is easy.

Indeed, it is surprisingly easy and what so many find so much more surprising still is the fact that this is not head-hurting school learning at all but exciting, fun, stimulating, sexy, funny, breath-takingly amazing and on occasion frighteningly exciting, too.

And that IS our first lesson in quantum logic – FORGET about learning being difficult or painful. FORGET THAT. That was learning the hard way and you can't learn hard amidst the flowing, glowing vibrant Oceans of Energy from which we came, and to which we will return in glory and delight, a homecoming of such wonder and awe, it will take your breath away.

For anyone seriously interested in getting really serious about learning, it's time to seriously lighten up and start learning for yourself, by yourself, in yourself – a one-on-one tuition between you and the universe itself. Project Sanctuary is your manual, handbook and tour guide - if you want it.

Project Sanctuary by Silvia Hartmann, PhD

ISBN 1 873483 98 8

Available from:

https://DragonRising.com

+44 (0)1323 729 666

Truly Revolutionary Energy Hypnosis

The HypnoDreams Trilogy

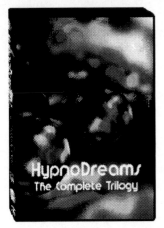

Energy alignment experiences for the conscious mind, the energy mind, the body and the energy body plus stimulation for your neurology and for your psychic circuitry – or simply, lay back, relax and travel far away, into the states of beauty and of freedom, wonder and expansion.

This fantastic collection contains the entire HypnoDreams trilogy, designed, created and delivered by Silvia Hartmann and with original sonic solutions sound tracks by Ananga Sivyer, PLUS the amazing "Our Dimensions" accompanying eBook on data CD.

The Wisdom of The Water – *High Quality Stereo Hypnosis Audio CD*

Heart Healing - *High Quality Stereo Hypnosis Audio CD*

Freedom – *High Quality Stereo Hypnosis Audio CD*

Plus **Our Dimensions** – *The HypnoDreams Guide & Script Book – Data CD*

Awaken The Psychic Circuitry with:

The Appollonius Quartet

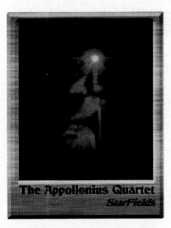

Improve psychic abilities, paranormal skills and enhance and restore the psychic circuitry with this revolutionary and advanced energy hypnosis programme.

This programme consists of four different yet parallel inductions and it comes complete with accompanying scripts book, instructions for usage and additional information about psychic circuitry enhancement. The Appollonius Quartet Program:

The Lighthouse, Journey Of Your Soul, Night Eyes, Magic Of The Day Plus Instruction Ebook Energy Hypnosis Programs

For You, A Star

Essential Magic For Every Day

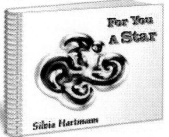

55 Positive, Magical Essences – positive energies to lift, raise, heal and inspire.

No work to do - just pick your Essence, look at the image, read the evocaton, take a deep breath and move away from every day stress, from trouble and strife – open up and contact the calm and healing energy of your Essence of choice!

A pure and wonderful application of the principles of high "Energy Magic" created for you by Silvia Hartmann – this is a buffet for your soul.

The Enchanted World

Welcome To The Wonderworlds Of Energy!

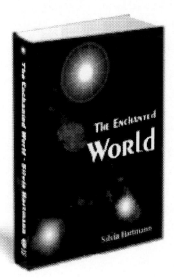

Over 25 years in the making – The Enchanted World is Silvia Hartmann's introduction, overview and invitation to begin to explore the wonderworlds of energy.

Energy is everywhere – it is all around us and behind each and every action we take, each object we own and each word that we speak.

Without an understanding of these amazing realms, life simply doesn't make any sense; but when we re-connect with The Enchanted World, everything changes.

The possibilities for change, for healing and for growth, for discovery and for sheer joy of living, life and love of life come back to us and are once more, available to each and every one of us. This book is a gift to all.

The Enchanted World

by Silvia Hartmann - ISBN 1873483 57 0

Available from

https://DragonRising.com

+44 (0)1323 729 666

About DragonRising

DragonRising is an International Publisher of high quality books, courses, events, audio CDs & trainings in the fields of EmoTrance, Emotional Freedom Techniques (EFT), Ayurveda, Creativity and Magic.

Working with cutting-edge authors and presenters at the forefront of our fields, DragonRising has helped thousands of people around the world to learn more about these 21st century modalities and therapeutic techniques.

To find out more about us, please visit our website:

https://DragonRising.com

You'll find our latest news, reviews, product samples free to download, information for affiliates & resellers and our online shop.

We love to hear from our customers so if you have any reviews, opinions, criticisms, praise & suggestions then we'd love to hear from you.

If you haven't got access to a computer and still want to stay in touch then we have an offline mailing list & news letter. To add yourself, write to the following address requesting to be included:

DragonRising
18 Marlow Avenue
Eastbourne
East Sussex
BN22 8SJ
United Kingdom
Tel: +44 (0)1323 729 666

Energy Magic – The Patterns & Techniques of EmoTrance, Vol 3

First Edition

All Patterns & Articles © Silvia Hartmann 2002/2006.

All Rights Reserved In All Media.